NUTRITION AND DIET RESEARCH PROGRESS

APRICOTS AND PEACHES

NUTRITIONAL PROPERTIES, POST-HARVEST MANAGEMENT AND POTENTIAL HEALTH BENEFITS

NUTRITION AND DIET RESEARCH PROGRESS

Additional books in this series can be found on Nova's website under the Series tab.

Additional e-books in this series can be found on Nova's website under the e-book tab.

NUTRITION AND DIET RESEARCH PROGRESS

APRICOTS AND PEACHES

NUTRITIONAL PROPERTIES, POST-HARVEST MANAGEMENT AND POTENTIAL HEALTH BENEFITS

JEANNE HANSEN
EDITOR

nova publishers
New York

Library of Congress Cataloging-in-Publication Data

ISBN: 978-1-63484-684-4

Library of Congress Control Number: 2016930410

Published by Nova Science Publishers, Inc. † New York

CONTENTS

PREFACE

This book presents research on the nutritional properties, post-harvest management and potential health benefits of apricots and peaches. Chapter One provides a brief description of the production area of wild apricot in India, the nutritional properties and health benefits of wild apricot, and the useful products made from the fruit. Chapter Two summarizes the current knowledge on Japanese apricot, including its correlation with oral diseases for preventive medicine. Chapter Three discusses properties, deficit irrigation strategies and post-harvest management of peaches and nectarines. Chapter Four reviews the impact of different industrial processing techniques of sterilization and associated storage conditions on nutritional and functional characteristics of the processed peach, and establishes their role on the nutritional and functional quality of fruit. Chapter Five examines the physico-chemical and sensory characterization of Sicilian white flesh peaches.

Chapter 1 - Wild apricot locally called Chullu is found in abundance in the dry temperate regions of Himachal Pradesh and Uttarakhand and particularly in the valleys of Kashmir, Chenab, and Kulu, Simla and Garhwal hills at altitudes up to 2500 m. Fruit is harvested from May to July. It is highly perishable. Apricot is a good source of sugars and vitamin A and contains appreciable amounts of thiamine and iron. Fresh Indian apricots yield 86 percent of edible matter which contains total solids 12.4 to 16.7%, insoluble solids 2.1 to 3.1%, malic acid 0.7 to 2.2%, total sugars 5.3 to 8.6%. The wild apricot is unfit for table purpose due to its high acid and low sugar content. It is not processed for any commercial product at present. Some studies for preparation of sauces and chutney from this fruit has given quite encouraging results. The major portion of the crop is utilized by the tribal in Himachal Pradesh for the preparation of distilled alcoholic liquor. The wild apricot pits yield 22 to 38 percent kernels, which may be used as its substitute in pastes and confectionery and can be added to apricot jams. The fatty oil extracted from the apricot kernels is an important article of commerce. It is also source of an essential oil identical with that obtained from bitter almond cake. The apricot kernel oil is used for food purposes and in cosmetics and pharmaceutical preparations. It sells at a higher price than most food oils. The cake left after pressing out oil is used as manure or fuel. This chapter deals with the brief description of production area of wild apricot in India, nutritional Properties and health benefits of wild apricot and the useful products production from it.

Chapter 2 - The oral cavity is inhabited by over 500 different bacterial species. Dental caries and periodontitis are major bacterial infectious diseases in the oral cavity.

Prunus mume Sieb. et Zucc., which is a variety of Japanese apricot known as *Ume* in Japanese, has been a traditional Japanese medicine for centuries and is a familiar and commonly consumed food. The health benefits of *Ume* are now being widely recognized. Recent studies showed that MK615, an extract of compounds from *Ume*, has strong anticancer and anti-inflammatory effects. However, the potential role of MK615 in the oral field remains unknown. The authors herein demonstrate that MK615 significantly reduced the production of pro-inflammatory mediators (tumor necrosis factor-alpha, interleukin(IL)-6, and IL-8) induced by *Porphyromonas gingivalis* lipopolysaccharide (LPS), a major etiological agent in localized chronic periodontitis. Moreover, the authors show that MK615 may be a potent inhibitor of the growth of some oral bacteria and an inhibitor of biofilm formation by *Streptococcus mutans*, the principal etiological agent of human dental caries. The authors' findings suggest that MK615 has potential as a therapeutic agent for treating and preventing oral diseases such as periodontitis and dental caries.

This review summarizes the current knowledge on Japanese apricot, including its correlation with oral diseases for preventive medicine.

Chapter 3 - Nowadays, Spain is the fourth largest producer of nectarine and peach with an average annual volume of 1,219,780.50 tonnes. This quantity has increased in recent years due to the new varieties obtained which are adapted to each geographical area and specific soil conditions. Also, it is due to advances in irrigation and fertilization strategies, as well as improvements in postharvest techniques and traceability that promote export opportunities. Stone fruit crops require an average of 5,000 to 7,000 m^3 of irrigation water per hectare and year. In Mediterranean areas or the southern of the United States, great nectarine and peach producers, agriculture is limited by scarce water supplies and their poor quality. Therefore, the application of irrigation strategies to optimize water use, but maintain yield and quality is essential. These techniques are generally known as regulated deficit irrigation (RDI). Their use assumes knowledge of each crop phenological stage in order to avoid possible adverse effects on both plant growth and fruit. In recent years, consumers have increasingly requested products with high sensory, microbiological and nutritional quality. Consumers are also interested in purchasing products grown under sustainable techniques. Currently, there is also an increasing interest in the consumption of fruits and vegetables with high antioxidant potential. That is to say, commodities that contain health-promoting compounds, such as vitamin C and certain individual polyphenols. Previous studies have observed an increase in these biocompounds when the product has been subjected to RDI. This is caused by the activation of specific metabolic pathways that lead to the synthesis of these biocompounds as a response to water stress. In this chapter, the production and characteristics of peaches and nectarines are contextualized. Here, the main effects of deficit irrigation on fruit quality and bioactive compounds during peach and nectarine growth and postharvest period have been taken into account. Postharvest management of these commodities either as whole product or minimally processed is explained, listing the main recommendations.

Chapter 4 - Peach is a fruit with high content of phytochemical compounds with antioxidant activity, namely polyphenols and carotenes that make them a healthy fruit for consumers. Peach (*Prunus persica* (L.)), is an important commercial Mediterranean fruit during summer season not only for its high water content, fibre and minerals, but also for its high content in antioxidant molecules such as procyanidins, anthocyanins, catechins, phenolic acids and carotenoids (lutein, zeaxanthin, β-cryptoxanthin and β-carotene). These compounds in peach fruit vary strongly in relation to different environmental and agricultural factors, such as cultivar, rootstock, water and ripening stage at harvest.

Besides the regular peach consumption as fresh fruit, processed products such as juices, jams, jellies, smoothies, canned fruit and others, are usually produced from fruit fresh market.

Information about nutrient content of processed fruits is of interest to consumers as they are becoming more aware and interested about their related health benefits. Fruit processing and storage may lead to negative or positive effects concerning their nutritional value according the processing steps they are exposed to. There are occurrences during fruit processing where chemical reactions could release bound components leading to a promotion of nutritional quality.

Among the phytochemicals, phenols, have received a great deal of attention because of their antioxidant activity, which help to neutralise free radicals. Thermal treatment is one of the most important factors affecting their stability. Previous studies have shown that concentrations of carotenoids often increase during heat treatment, probably because cell walls are softened, making the extraction of carotenoids easier during analysis. Extreme or prolonged heat treatment, however, enhances loss of carotenoids. Factors such as light, metals, oxygen, organic acids and heat can promote carotenoid isomerization and degradation.

The aim of this chapter, therefore, is to review the impact of different industrial processing techniques of sterilization and associated storage conditions (e.g., time and temperature) on nutritional and functional characteristics of processed peach, and to establish their role on the nutritional and functional quality of fruit.

Chapter 5 - *Pescabivona* [*Prunus persica* (L.) Batch] is the name of an autochthonous peach population of the Middle-West of Sicily. Samples of the four *Pescabivona* landraces (*Murtiddara*, *Bianca*, *Agostina*, and *Settembrina*) were harvested at three different altitudes and analysed for chemical, physico-chemical, and sensory descriptors. The data obtained have supported the application for registration of *Pescabivona* as Protected Geographical Indication (P.G.I.).

Statistic data processing outlined a substantial match in the composition of the four landraces at the different altitudes, highlighting high values of flesh firmness corresponding to balanced sugar/acidity ratios, in particular for the late ripening landraces (*Agostina* and *Settembrina*). In addition, a large content of lactones (the key odorant molecules) was found. A good agreement between sensory evaluation and composition was observed. In particular, the sensory liking was correlated with the main ripeness parameters, as well as with the pulp firmness.

Therefore, in periods of the year when the quality of the peaches is generally decreasing, the chance of tasting firm fruits at physiological ripeness and with a pleasant sensory profile as showed by *Pescabivona* is not very common.

In: Apricots and Peaches
Editor: Jeanne Hansen
ISBN: 978-1-63484-684-4

Chapter 1

APRICOT: PRODUCTION, NUTRITIONAL PROPERTIES, HEALTH BENEFITS AND POST-HARVEST UTILIZATION: AN OVERVIEW

Anwesa Sarkar, A. E. Kate, Anupama Singh and N. C. Shahi

Department of Post Harvest Process and Food Engineering, College of Technology G. B. Pant University of Agriculture and Technology, Pantnagar, Uttarakhand, India

ABSTRACT

Wild apricot locally called Chullu is found in abundance in the dry temperate regions of Himachal Pradesh and Uttarakhand and particularly in the valleys of Kashmir, Chenab, and Kulu, Simla and Garhwal hills at altitudes up to 2500 m. Fruit is harvested from May to July. It is highly perishable. Apricot is a good source of sugars and vitamin A and contains appreciable amounts of thiamine and iron. Fresh Indian apricots yield 86 percent of edible matter which contains total solids 12.4 to 16.7%, insoluble solids 2.1 to 3.1%, malic acid 0.7 to 2.2%, total sugars 5.3 to 8.6%. The wild apricot is unfit for table purpose due to its high acid and low sugar content. It is not processed for any commercial product at present. Some studies for preparation of sauces and chutney from this fruit has given quite encouraging results. The major portion of the crop is utilized by the tribal in Himachal Pradesh for the preparation of distilled alcoholic liquor. The wild apricot pits yield 22 to 38 percent kernels, which may be used as its substitute in pastes and confectionery and can be added to apricot jams. The fatty oil extracted from the apricot kernels is an important article of commerce. It is also source of an essential oil identical with that obtained from bitter almond cake. The apricot kernel oil is used for food purposes and in cosmetics and pharmaceutical preparations. It sells at a higher price than most food oils. The cake left after pressing out oil is used as manure or fuel. This chapter deals with the brief description of production area of wild apricot in India, nutritional Properties and health benefits of wild apricot and the useful products production from it.

1. Introduction

The wild apricot (Prunus armeniaca Linn.) is an important tree borne oilseed of mid hills and dry temperate regions of India. Wild apricot belong to the family Rosaceae and sub-family Prunoidea. In the Himalayan region of the country, local communities known it by different vernacular names viz. "Chulli," "Shara," "Khurmani," "Chulu," "Aaroo" Zardhi, Khubani, Chuari, Kushmiaru, Chola and Gurdulu. In Punjabi, it is called as Hari, Sari and Chuli.

2. Production

The cultivated apricot has its origin in North-Eastern China, whereas, wild apricot appears to be indigenous to India. In India wild apricot locally called Chullu is found in the dry temperate regions of North-Western Himalayas particularly in the valleys of Jammu and Kashmir (especially Ladakh), Chenab; Kullu and Shimla regions of H.P. and Garhwal hills of Uttrakhand at altitudes up to 3000 m. In Kumaon region, wild apricot is found in all the three districts of Nainital, Almora and Pithoragarh. Pithorgarh district has maximum density of wild apricot tree in the Kumaon region.

The wild apricot tree is about 10-15 m tall with a reddish brown bark. Leaves are ovate to round, approximately 5-9 cm long. Its somatic chromosome number is (2 n) 16 and basic chromosome number (X), is 8. Flowers are solitary, white or pinkish, about 2.5 cm across, borne singly and appearing much in advance of the foliage. Fruits are around 1.5-4.0 cm across or more and hairy when young but nearly smooth skinned at maturity. The appearances of the fruits are yellowish with light red cheek and nearly glabrous. The flesh is yellow or yellowish orange to firm and sweet. Stone is smooth with a thickened furrowed edge.

Wild apricot is quite hardy and can be grown in most of the soils, which are deep and well drained. The horizontal and vertical root distribution of a ten year old tree reached 4.5 and 2.2 metre, respectively indicating that the soil for wild apricot should be about 3 m deep. The tree growing in wet soil can depress physiological activity of leaves and overall the growth of the plant. In Kinnaur district of Himachal Pradesh where it is grown in large area, the soils are sandy, well drained but not very fertile. The pH of the soil should be 6.0-6.8. Wild apricot thrives best in mid hills at elevations of 1200-3000 m above mean sea level. The long cool winter (800 chilling hours below 70 C), and frostfree and warm spring are favorable for fruiting. Average summer temperature (16.6°C–32.3°C) is suitable for better growth and quality fruit production. The sites located in north-eastern India at lower elevations and on south-western at higher elevations are also suitable for its cultivations. Spring frost causes extensive damage to the blossoms, which are killed when temperature falls below 40 C.

An annual rainfall of about 100 cm well distributed throughout the season is good for its normal growth and fruiting. Wild apricot trees are usually grown under rain fed conditions. Being a hardy plant and tolerant to dry atmosphere, no additional irrigation is required by the trees. But application of irrigation water during the dry spell of summer months facilitate the establishment of the young plants and improves the flowering and fruiting of the well grown trees.

Wild apricot fruits generally start maturing from last week of May and continue upto August end depending upon altitude and location. They are harvested manually by shaking the tree branches and no mechanical harvesting is practiced. Change of surface colour, days from full bloom to harvesting and fruit total sugar solids (TSS) are considered as the best indices of maturity. For fresh marketing, fruits should be plucked when they change their surface colour from green to yellow. Fully ripe fruits are harvested for freezing, canning and drying. The fruits should be harvested in morning hours and direct exposure of fruits to sun should be avoided during grading and packaging. Tree starts bearing at the age of 4-5 years and continues to bear well for 50- 60 years. The full bearing occurs at about 10-15 years when it yields about 85-100 kg. fruits per tree. The stone yield varies from 12-17 percent of fruits and the kernel yield ranges 3.14-4.81 kg/tree. The yield of a full-bearing well maintained tree varies from 120-150 kg.

Table 1. Ripe fruit pulp contents of wild apricot fruit

Total solids 12.4	16.7 percent
Insoluble solids 2.1	3.1 percent
Acids (as malic acid) 0.7	2.2 percent
Total sugars (as invert sugar) 5.3	8.6 percent
Glucose 3.2	4.8 percent
Fructose 1.4	4.25 percent
Sucrose 1.4	5.4 percent
Tannin 0.06	0.10 percent

3. Nutritional Properties

Apricot is a good source of sugars and Vitamin A and contains appreciable amounts of thiamine and iron. Fresh wild apricots yield 86 percent of edible matter, which contain following elements:

The wild apricot fruits yield 22-38 percent kernels, which may be sweet or bitter depending on the type. Sweet kernels resemble almonds in taste and are used as its substitute in pastes and confectionery and can be added to apricot jams. The kernels contains Water (4.3%), Protein (31.4%), Oil (53.4%), Fiber (4.8%), Ash (2.6%) Sugar direct (8.1%) and as dextrose after conversion (11.6%)Kernel oil closely resembles expressed almond oil thus it is employed as an adulterant or a substitute for almond oil. The cake after extraction of oil contains Nitrogen (6.64%), Phosphoric acid (2.2%), Potash (1.14%) An essential oil that is identical with bitter almond oil is distilled from the cake. Apricot kernels are cheaper and give higher yield of oil (0.8 – 1.6 percent) than bitter almond oil. The seed cake of the bitter apricot yields 1.6 percent of the oil. The cake from which the oil has been removed is free of hydrocyanic acid and can be used as a feed stuff for livestock.

4. Health Benefits and Post Harvest Utilisation

The wild apricot is unfit for table purpose due to high acids and low sugars. It is not processed for any commercial product at present although studies for preparation of sauces and chutney from this fruit have given quite encouraging results. The major portion of the crop pulp is utilized by the tribals in Himachal Pradesh and Uttrakhand for the preparation of distilled alcoholic liquor. The fruits are highly perishable and can be preserved in a number of ways. They are frozen, candied or made into a paste. In some countries, fruit pulp is cooked and thinly spread on cloth and then rolled and dried and it constitutes an important food. A number of products are prepared from fruits of apricot. Its fruits mixed with those of cultivated types are utilized in Himachal Pradesh in production of number of products like apricot jam, apricot nectar, and apricot papad. The strained baby foods from pulp is nutritious and a good source of calcium, phosphorus and iron. The oil of seed is edible and oil cake can be used as organic manure.

The health benefits of apricot include its ability to treat indigestion, constipation, earaches, fevers, skin diseases, cancer and anemia. Apricot oil is useful for treating strained muscles and wounds. It is also believed that apricot is good for skin care, especially for women. This is why one can find it added in various cosmetics. Furthermore, apricots have the ability to improve heart health, reduce cholesterol levels, prevent the deterioration of vision, help to lose weight, treat respiratory conditions, boost bone strength, and maintain electrolyte balance in the body. The impressive health benefits of apricots are due to the content of vitamins, including vitamins A, C, K, E, and niacin in significant amounts, as well as a number of other essential vitamins in trace amounts (less than 5% of daily requirement), as well as their mineral content, which includes potassium, copper manganese, magnesium, and phosphorous. Apricots are also a very good source of dietary fiber, like most fruits.

Apricot kernel oil is obtained from the kernels (seeds) of Apricots. After eating these delicious fruits, the seeds are used to make this light oil. Apricot kernel oil is great for use as a massage oil as it is very light and makes the skin soft. Apricot kernels themselves are quite healthy and are being researched for a number of health conditions including cancer. Apricot kernel oil is quite similar to almond oil and its applications are also similar. This oil has a deep, nutty flavor which makes it an excellent ingredient for desserts and other recipes.

Apricot oil is really a rich source of fatty acids in addition to Vitamin E and A. Therefore it is very theraputic for dealing with dry as well as mature skin and keep the skin revitalized. In case your skin feels scratchy or dry after having a bath, use this oil in your damp skin and you'll get relief. This oil is a crucial ingredient in lots of the cosmetics just like soaps, creams as well as skin lotions. It gets absorbed within the skin fast and doesn't make the skin oily. Therefore, lots of people prefer it for massaging the body and also as sunbathing oil on the beach. Massaging the body with this particular oil works well for eliminating stress, pain and inflammation. Being mild as well as nonirritating, additionally it is great for massaging infants and children. It could also be added like a base in lots of aromatherapy oils too. Usage of apricot kernel oil could be healthier for the heart and also the cardiovascular system. This oil has revealed capability to lower the chance of myocardial infarction (heart attack) in rats and may possibly perform the same function in humans. One can take apricot oil in food like a salad dressing and by utilizing it for cooking particular recipes that go well with all the flavor of the oil.

Besides its use as a healing agent along with a home cure for skincare, apricot kernel oil has numerous more uses. It really is utilized in some recipes exactly where it really brings out better flavor. However it is usually used only like a salad dressing regularly. Moreover, it has also got some industrial applications. Apricot oil is utilized just as one component in soaps. Additionally it is an excellent carrier for essential oils that are utilized in soap making like lemon essential oil, lavender oil as well as jasmine essential oil. Apricot kernel oil is being examined because of its possibility to generate biodiesel and also the results so far look good. Particularly the oil from wild apricot varieties bring this purpose. The nutritional value of 1 cup of apricot kernel oil is given in Table 2.

Table 2. Nutritional Information of Apricot Seed Oil

Nutrients	Amount
Calories from Fat	1927
Monounsaturatedfat	131 g
Omega 6-Fatty acids	63872 mg
Phytolesterols	580 g
Polyunsaturated fat	63.9 g
Protein	1.4 g
Saturated Fat	13.7 g
Vitamin E	8.7 g

Side Effects, Safety and Toxicity Issues

Apricot kernel oil is usually secure topically. However, whenever utilized internally, there is one thing to note. Apricot kernels include a substance known as amygdalin. This really is converted by the body into cyanide, that is poisonous. This may lead to respiratory failure and may also be fatal. Amygdalin is generally removed from oil products. This is done to make sure that the oil product contains much less amygdalin than the safety limit. This is actually the case with almond oil, apricot oil and peach oil. However, one should be absolutely sure that the oil product have been processed to eliminate this poisonous substance.

REFFERENCES

[1] Kureel, R. S., Singh, C. B.,Gupta, A. K. and Pandey, Ashutosh.(2007). *WILD APRICOT National Oilseeds and Vegetable Oils Development Board.*

[2] Hegedus, A., Engel, R., Abranko, L., Balogh, E., Blazovics, A., Herman, R., Halasz, J., Ercisli, S., Pedryc, A. and Stefanovits-Banyai, E. (2010). Antioxidant and antiradical capacities in apricot (Prunus armeniaca L.) fruits: Variation from genotypes, years, and analytical methods. *J Food Sci*, *75*(9), C722–C730.

[3] Hegedus, A., Pfeiffer, P., Papp, N., Abranko, L., Blazovics, A., Pedryc, A. and Stefanovits-Banyai, E. (2011). Accumulation of antioxidants in apricot fruit through Kan et al. Biological Research 2014, 47:46 Page 5 of 6 http://www.biolres.com/content/47/1/46 ripening: characterization of a genotype with enhanced functional properties. *Biol Res*, *44*, 339–344.

[4] Kim, D. O., Jeong, S. W. and Lee, C. Y. (2003). Antioxidant capacity of phenolic phytochemicals from various cultivars of plums. *Food Chem*,*81*, 321–326.

[5] Health Benefits of Apricots. (2015). https://www.organicfacts.net/health-benefits/fruit/apricots.html.

[6] Apricot Kernel Oil. (2015). http://oilhealthbenefits.com/apricot-kernel-oil/.

In: Apricots and Peaches
Editor: Jeanne Hansen

ISBN: 978-1-63484-684-4

Chapter 2

JAPANESE APRICOT (*UME*): POTENTIAL ORAL HEALTH BENEFITS

Yoko Morimoto-Yamashita, Masayuki Tokuda and Yoshihiro Nishitani

Department of Restorative Dentistry and Endodontology, Kaogoshima University Graduate School of Medical and Dental Sciences, Sakuragaoka, Kagoshima, Japan

ABSTRACT

The oral cavity is inhabited by over 500 different bacterial species. Dental caries and periodontitis are major bacterial infectious diseases in the oral cavity.

Prunus mume Sieb. et Zucc., which is a variety of Japanese apricot known as *Ume* in Japanese, has been a traditional Japanese medicine for centuries and is a familiar and commonly consumed food. The health benefits of *Ume* are now being widely recognized. Recent studies showed that MK615, an extract of compounds from *Ume*, has strong anticancer and anti-inflammatory effects. However, the potential role of MK615 in the oral field remains unknown. We herein demonstrate that MK615 significantly reduced the production of pro-inflammatory mediators (tumor necrosis factor-alpha, interleukin(IL)-6, and IL-8) induced by *Porphyromonas gingivalis* lipopolysaccharide (LPS), a major etiological agent in localized chronic periodontitis. Moreover, we show that MK615 may be a potent inhibitor of the growth of some oral bacteria and an inhibitor of biofilm formation by *Streptococcus mutans*, the principal etiological agent of human dental caries. Our findings suggest that MK615 has potential as a therapeutic agent for treating and preventing oral diseases such as periodontitis and dental caries.

This review summarizes the current knowledge on Japanese apricot, including its correlation with oral diseases for preventive medicine.

INTRODUCTION

Many fruits contain nutrient substances that can prevent, cure or suppress various diseases. They are nature's true medicines, and diets rich in fruits are consistently associated with a decreased risk of cancer and other chronic diseases. Apricot, *Prunus armeniaca*, is the fruit of a rosaceous tree (Rosaceae), which is produced in most parts of the world [1]. The name *Prunus armeniaca* is thought to be a misnomer based upon the long-held view that apricots initially originated in Armenia. It is known that apricots originated in the Far East, most likely in the Himalayas, the Northern and Western regions of China from where they spread to Armenia and Russia [2, 3]. Apricots are found semi-wild and wild in the northern hills of China and in a broad belt across the hills, mountains, and plateaus of Central Asia as far as the Caucasus Mountains. The first record of the domestication of apricots is an account of their cultivation in China, approximately 4,000 years ago. It is likely that tribe people of Central Asia established traditional rights to harvest their parts of the apricot forests for millennia before this time.

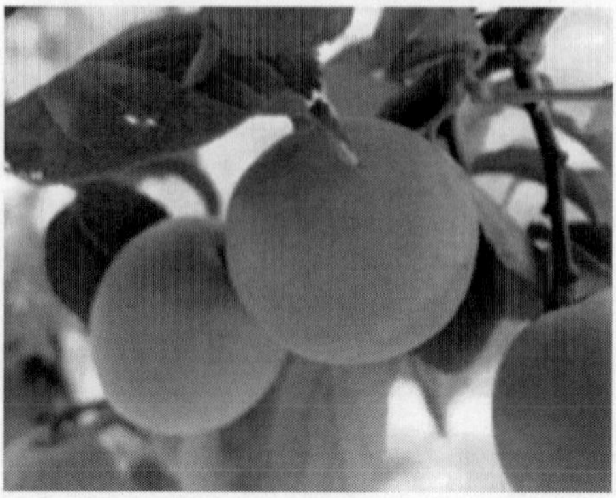

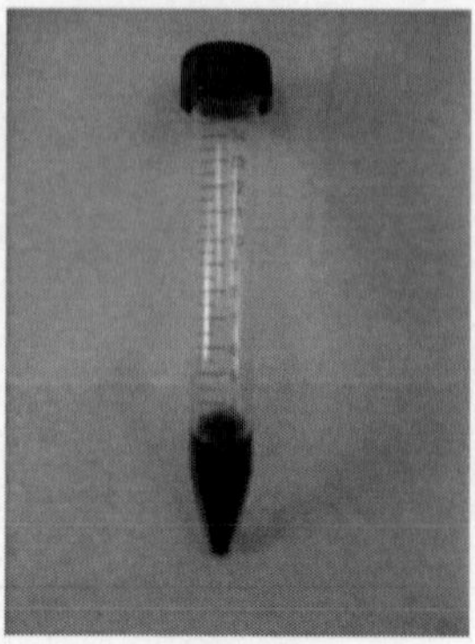

Japanese apricot fruits MK615

Figure 1. MK615 is extracted from Japanese apricot (*Ume*).

The apricot variety found in Japan is *Prunus mume Sieb. et Zucc*, widely known as *Ume* (Figure 1). The Japanese people started to grow *Ume* trees more than 2,000 years ago, most likely imported from China. They soon discovered the health enhancing effects of apricot fruits, and over many centuries, through cultivation, they have improved the apricot tree variety to produce healthier fruits. Accordingly, there is a long-standing view that the Japanese apricot juice can suppress cancer in tumor-bearing hosts and inhibit the growth of bacteria.

This review summarizes the current knowledge on the Japanese apricot, including its correlation with disease and preventive medicine.

Anti-Cancer Effects of an Extract from *Ume*

MK615 is a compound extracted from the Japanese apricot *Prunus mume* (AdaBio, Gunma, Japan) and contains several triterpenoids, such as oleanolic acid and ursolic acid [4]. It has been reported that MK615 inhibits cell growth and induces the death of several tumor cell lines, including gastric cancer [5], promyelocytic leukemia [5], breast cancer [6], pancreatic cancer [7], hepatocellular carcinoma [8, 9], colon cancer [10], malignant melanoma [11, 12] and lung cancer cells [13]. The activities underlying the anti-tumor effects of MK615 have been reported to include the induction of apoptosis [5, 6], autophagy [10, 13] and the suppression of aurora A kinase [7, 8]. Furthermore, some clinical studies have shown promising effects in some cancer patients [5, 10]. Recently, hepatoprotective effects of MK615 have been reported for patients with chronic liver diseases [14].

Inhibitory Effects of an Extract from *Ume* on *Helicobacter Pylori*

Helicobacter pylori infection is an important factor in human gastric disorders, including chronic active gastritis, peptic ulcers, intestinal metaplasia and cancer.

In an *in vitro* study, *Ume* extract had an immediate bactericidal effect on *H. pylori* [15, 16]. In an *in vivo* study, *Ume* extract suppressed chronic active gastritis in the glandular stomachs of *H. pylori*-infected Mongolian gerbils [17]. *H. pylori*-inoculated gerbils were given *Ume* extract in their drinking water for 10 weeks. The microscopic scores for gastritis and mucosal hyperplasia in the *Ume* extract groups were significantly lower than that of the *H. pylori*-inoculated control group, with a dose-dependent response. Additionally, it was reported that *Ume* extract showed an antibacterial effect on *H. pylori* in a human stomach *in vivo* pilot study [18]. Therefore, *Ume* extract may be a potentially safe and inexpensive agent to control *H. pylori*-associated gastric disorders, including gastric neoplasia.

Anti-Inflammatory Effects of MK615

The high mobility group box 1 protein (HMGB1), a nuclear protein, has two distinct functions in cellular systems. In the nucleus, HMGB1 acts as an intracellular regulator of the transcription process with a crucial role in the maintenance of DNA functions [19]. In the extracellular space, HMGB1 is released by all eukaryotic cells upon necrosis or by various cells in response to inflammatory stimuli, such as endotoxins, tumor necrosis factor (TNF)-α, and C-reactive protein [20-22]. Extracellular HMGB1 can act as a potent inducer of proinflammatory cytokines including TNF-α, interleukin (IL)-6, and IL-1 from various cell types, thus playing a major role in various inflammatory diseases such as sepsis, rheumatoid arthritis, periodontitis and atherosclerosis [20, 21, 23-25]. Therefore, agents capable of inhibiting HMGB1 can be considered to possess therapeutic potential.

We previously reported that an extract of *Ume*, an abundant source of triterpenoids, strongly inhibited HMGB1 release from lipopolysaccharide (LPS)-stimulated macrophage-like RAW264.7 cells [4]. The inhibitory effect on HMGB1 release was enhanced by pure oleanolic acid, a naturally occurring triterpenoid. Similarly, the HMGB1 release inhibitor in *Ume* extract was found to be oleanolic acid. Regarding the mechanisms of the inhibition of HMGB1 release, oleanolic acid or *Ume* extract was found to activate the transcription factor Nrf2, which binds to the antioxidative responsive element, and subsequently the heme oxygenase (HO)-1 protein was induced, indicating that the inhibition of HMGB1 release from LPS-stimulated RAW264.7 cells was mediated via the Nrf2/HO-1 system, an essential antioxidant effect. These results suggested that natural sources of triterpenoids warrant further evaluation as “rescue” therapeutics for sepsis and other potentially fatal systemic inflammatory disorders.

ORAL DISEASES

Periodontal Disease

Periodontal disease, which includes gingivitis and periodontitis, is the most common chronic disorder of infectious origin known in humans, with a prevalence of 10–60% in adults depending on the diagnostic criteria used [26]. Periodontitis is a chronic inflammatory disease of which the primary etiological factor is microbial dental plaque which causes an inflammatory response [27]. Periodontitis is initiated by the overgrowth of specific Gram-negative anaerobic bacteria, including *Aggregatibacter actionmycetem-comitans* and *Porphyromonas gingivalis*, which leads to the gingival inflammation characteristic of localized aggressive or chronic periodontitis. Recently, the LPSs of *A. actinomycetemcomitans* and *P. gingivalis* were shown to contribute to the processes leading to alveolar bone loss and connective tissue destruction in periodontitis [28-30]. The LPSs of Gram-negative bacteria are potent inducers of pro-inflammatory mediators and can initiate a number of host-mediated destructive processes [31]. Moreover, the continuously elevated secretion of various cytokines, including TNF-α, IL-6 and IL-8, by host cells following stimulation with periodontal pathogens and their products is a critical determinant of periodontal tissue destruction [32, 33]. The cytokines produced by LPS-activated macrophages or/and other cells are also potent inducers of inflammatory mediators, and have been identified as major mediators of inflammatory processes [34]. Therefore, blockade of cytokines secreted by LPS-stimulated cells may suppress proinflammatory responses and inhibit the development and progression of periodontal disease.

Periodontal Disease and Systemic Disease

In the last decade, many studies have been published indicating a positive relationship between periodontal disease and various systemic diseases. Significant associations between periodontal disease and cardiovascular disease, diabetes mellitus, preterm low birth weight and osteoporosis have been reported [35], bridging the once wide gap between medicine and dentistry. Researchers have hypothesized the etiologic role of periodontitis in the pathogenesis of these systemic diseases. Therefore, patients diagnosed with periodontal disease may be at a higher risk due to a compromised immune system as infectious and opportunistic microbes responsible for periodontal infection may prove a burden to the rest of the body. Furthermore, these microbes can release products that elicit an inflammatory response. Periodontal lesions are recognized as continually renewing reservoirs for the systemic spread of bacterial antigens, Gram-negative bacteria, cytokines and other proinflammatory mediators. Therefore, the development of new treatment modalities for periodontitis may contribute to the effective inhibition of systemic inflammatory diseases.

Dental Caries

Dental caries (tooth decay) is a major oral health problem in most industrialized countries, affecting 60–90% of schoolchildren and the vast majority of adults [36]. It is caused by specific bacteria (e.g., *Streptococcus mutans* and *S. sobrinus*). The bacteria build up on the teeth in a sticky film called plaque (dental biofilm) [37, 38]. This plaque also contains saliva, bits of food and other natural substances. *S. mutans* is the main pathogen for dental caries, although other acidogenic microorganisms may also be involved [39]. *S. mutans* produces three types of glucosyltransferase (GTFB, GTFC and GTFD) and synthesizes an adherent and water-insoluble glucan from sucrose that allows adherence of *S. mutans* to the tooth surface and dental plaque formation [40, 41]. The formation of a dental plaque biofilm leads to localized demineralization due to the accumulation of acids, thereby resulting in dental caries. The acids dissolve minerals in the hard enamel that covers the crown of the tooth. Theoretically, inhibition of each step in the process of caries formation will contribute to the prevention of dental caries [42].

Effects of MK615 on Oral Diseases

Anti-Inflammatory Effects of MK615

Natural compounds such as catechins in green tea, naringenin, a major flavanone in grapefruit, and polyphenols in cranberries may be useful for the prevention and treatment of inflammatory periodontal diseases [43-45]. Consequently, natural compounds with the capacity to modulate host inflammatory responses have received considerable attention, with the idea that they may be potential new therapeutic agents for the treatment of periodontal disease [46]. Some studies have indicated that MK615 may have not only anti-cancer effects, but also strong anti-inflammatory effects. MK615 contains several triterpenoids, including oleanolic acid and ursolic acid, and may have anti-inflammatory effects. Recent studies have suggested that triterpenoids have both anti-tumor and anti-inflammatory effects [4-8]. In the periodontal field, MK615 inhibits cytokine release, including that of TNF-α, IL-6 and IL-8 by *P. gingivalis* and *A. actinomycetemcomitans* LPS-stimulated cells in dose-dependent manners [47, 48]. These findings clearly indicate that MK615 contains an inhibitor of cytokine release. The continuously elevated secretion of various cytokines including TNF-α, IL-6 and IL-8 by host cells following stimulation with periodontal pathogens and their products is a critical determinant of periodontal tissue destruction. Therefore, blockade of TNF-α, IL-6 and IL-8 secreted by periodontal pathogens or other cytokines may suppress pro-inflammatory responses, and subsequently inhibit the development and progression of periodontal disease. It has been reported that LPS possibly induces the expression of TNF-α, IL-6 and IL-8 through transient phosphorylation of ERK1/2, JNK, and p38MAPK [49-53]. Additionally, it has been reported that the production of inflammatory cytokines requires nuclear factor kappaB (NF-κB) activation [54]. The inhibitory mechanism of MK615 is mediated by the attenuation of MAPK phosphorylation (Figure 2) and subsequent inactivation of NF-κB to suppress LPS-induced translocation and phosphorylation of the p65 subunit (Figure 3). These results support the notion that MK615 has anti-inflammatory effects, and MK615 may represent a key molecule with therapeutic potential for periodontitis. Therapeutic approaches that inhibit cytokine production are gaining increasing attention as potential options for managing chronic periodontitis.

Anti-Microbial Effects of MK615

Periodontitis and dental caries are major oral diseases. The formation of dental plaque, which plays an important role in the development of periodontal disease and caries in humans, can be initiated by several strains of oral streptococci [55, 56]. There is great interest in the use of antimicrobial agents for the prevention and treatment of periodontitis and caries. The prevention of periodontal disease and dental caries requires control of the pathogens that exist in the oral dental plaque biofilm. Chlorhexidine is a potent antiplaque chemical agent.

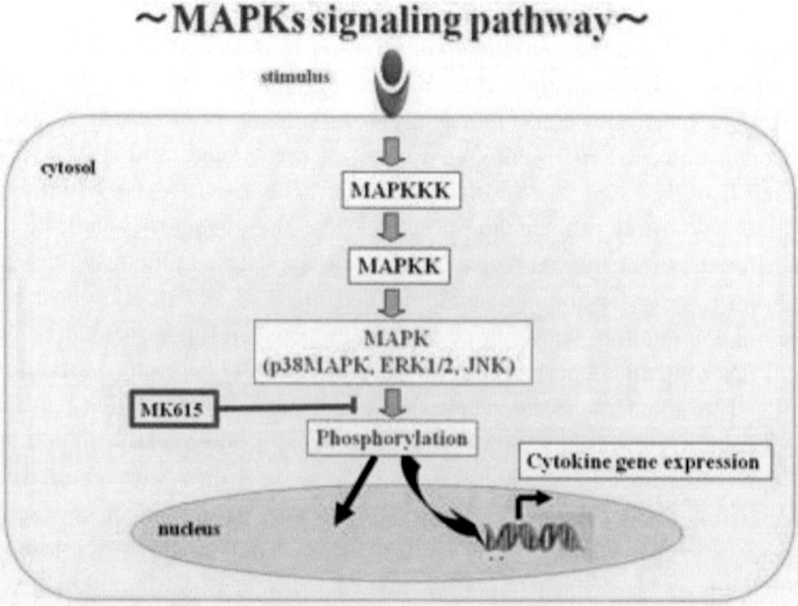

Figure 2. MK615 inhibits phosphorylation of MAPKs.

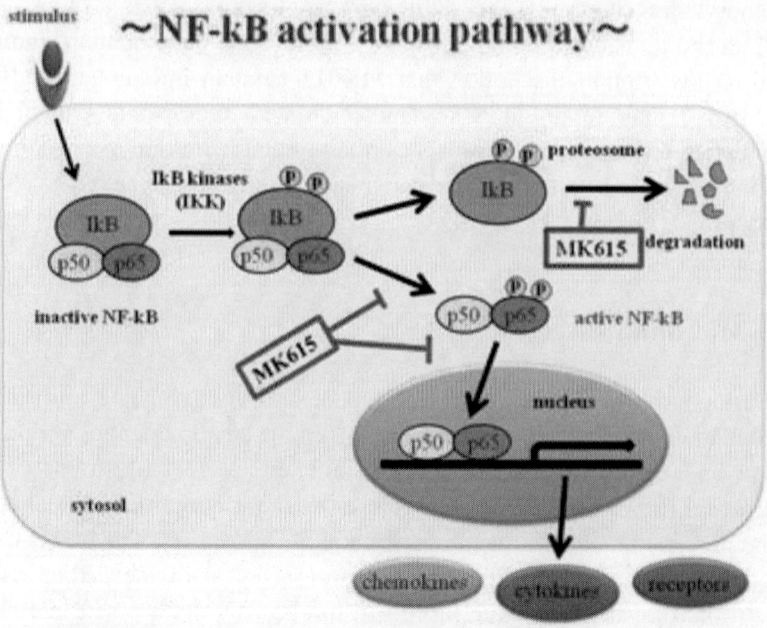

Figure 3. MK615 suppresses NF-κB activation but not degradation of IκB.

However, it has some side effects, such as altered taste sensation, desquamation and soreness of the oral mucosa [57]. Thus, it is important to develop alternative antiplaque agents from natural sources that have no side effects.

It has been reported that MK615 has not only anti-inflammatory effects for periodontal tissues, but also antimicrobial activity against periodontal bacteria, such as *A. actinomycetemcomitans* and *P. gingivalis*. In addition, MK615 exhibited antibacterial activity against cariogenic bacteria, such as *S. mutans*, *S. gordonii* and *S. sanguinis*, with an expected anti-caries effect (Table). Moreover, it was found that MK615 exhibited an inhibitory effect on *S. mutans* biofilm formation [58]. The most effective treatment against dental caries and periodontitis would be one that prevents early biofilm formation [59]. MK615 is known to contain active components with anti-inflammatory and anti-oxidative properties, such as oleanolic acid [4]. A previous study suggested that oleanolic acid has antimicrobial actions against *S. mutans* [60], while another study showed that oleanolic acid markedly inhibits water-insoluble glucan synthesis from sucrose by the crude glucosyltransferase of *S. mutans* [61]. Therefore, MK615 is a potential therapeutic agent for treating and preventing oral diseases such as periodontitis and dental caries. Further studies will focus on the active antimicrobial components in MK615, which should be identified and investigated for their mechanisms of action. Additionally, further studies are required to investigate the effects of local application of MK615 as an adjunctive treatment to conventional therapy for patients with periodontitis. Such studies may lead to the development of novel periodontal therapies and improved strategies for public oral health.

Table. MICs of MK615 against oral microorganisms

MICs of MK615 against oral microorganisms	
Species	(mg/ml)
A. actinomycetemcomitans 57	6.5
A. actinomycetemcomitans IDH	6.5
P. gingivalis	1.6
S. mutans UA159	13
S. mutans MT403R	13
S. mutans RIMD	13
S. gordonii	13
S. salivarius	(-)
S. sanguinis	13

CONCLUSION

With the growing recognition of their benefits for public health in recent years, natural foods are now being highlighted with special reference to their effects on human health in addition to their pharmacological actions. Japanese *Ume* has been used as an herbal medicine with several biological activities, including anticancer, antioxidant and anti-inflammatory effects [4-14].

MK615, an extract of compounds from Japanese *Ume*, has not only anti-inflammatory effects for periodontal tissues, but also antimicrobial activity against periodontal bacteria, such as *A. actinomycetemcomitans* and *P. gingivalis*. In addition, MK615 exhibited antibacterial activity against cariogenic bacteria, such as *S. mutans*, *S. gordonii* and *S. sanguinis*, with an anticipated anti-caries effect. Moreover, it was found that MK615 exhibited an inhibitory effect on *S. mutans* biofilm formation. Thus, MK615 is a potential therapeutic agent for treating and preventing oral diseases such as periodontitis and dental caries. Further studies will focus on the active anti-inflammatory and antimicrobial components in MK615, which should be identified and investigated for their mechanisms.

MK615 is safe in food for providing health benefits, and this remains unquestioned even when it is prescribed for oral therapy. Moreover, it is also used as a treatment for patients with liver cancer. In the future, it may be added to toothpastes, mouth rinses and other oral products that can be used easily by the majority of the population ranging from young children to the elderly. In addition, MK615 may be applicable to whole-body health through examining its potential effects on not only oral bacteria, but also *Staphylococcus aureus* and *Candida albicans*.

REFERENCES

[1] Gur AR., (1985). Deciduous Fruit Trees. In Handbook of Flowering. CRC Press., 355-389.

[2] Gu M., (1979). Apricot Cultivars in China. *Acta Horticulturae.*, 209, 63-67.

[3] Gulcan R., (1988). Apricot Cultivars in Near East. *Acta Horticulturae.*, 209, 49-54.

[4] Kawahara K., Hashiguchi T., Masuda K., Saniabadi AR., Kikuchi K., Tancharoen S., Ito T., Miura N., Morimoto Y., Biswas KK., Nawa Y.,

Meng X., Oyama Y., Takenouchi K., Shrestha B., Sameshima H., Shimizu T., Adachi T., Adachi M., Maruyama I., (2009). Mechanism of HMGB1 release inhibition from RAW264.7 cells by oleanolic acid in Prunus mume Sieb. et Zucc. *Int. J. Mol. Med.*, 23, 615-620.

[5] Adachi M., Suzuki Y., Mizuta T., Osawa T., Adachi T., Clerici M., (2007). The Japanese apricot *Prunus mume Sieb. et Zucc* (ume) is a rich natural source of novel anti-cancer substance. *Int J Food Prop.*, 10, 375-384.

[6] Nakagawa A., Sawada T., Okada T., Ohsawa T., Adachi M., Kubota K., (2007). New antineoplastic agent, MK615, from UME (a variety of) Japanese apricot inhibits growth of breast cancer cells in vitro. *Breast J.*, 13, 44-49.

[7] Okada T., Sawada T., Osawa T., Adachi M., Kubota K., (2008). MK615 inhibits pancreatic cancer cell growth by dual inhibition of Aurora A and B kinases. *World J Gastroenterol.*, 14, 1378-1382.

[8] Okada T., Sawada T., Osawa T., Adachi M., Kubota., (2007). A novel anti-cancer substance, MK615, from ume, a variety of Japanese apricot, inhibits growth of hepatocellular carcinoma cells by suppressing Aurora A kinase activity. *Hepato-gastroenterology.*, 54(78), 1770-1774.

[9] Hoshino T., Takagi H., Naganuma A., Koitabashi E., Uehara S., Sakamoto N., Kudo T., Sato K., Kakizaki S., (2013). Advanced hepatocellular carcinoma responds to MK615, a compound extract from the Japanese apricot "Prunus mume." *World J Hepatol.*, 5(10), 596-600.

[10] Mori S., Sawada T., Okada T., Ohsawa T., Adachi M., Keiichi K., (2007). New anti-proliferative agent, MK615, from Japanese apricot 'Prunus mume' induces striking autophagy in colon cancer cells in vitro. *World J Gastroenterol.*, 13, 6512-6517.

[11] Matsushita S., Tada KI., Kawahara KI., Kawai K., Hashiguchi T., Maruyama I., Kanekura T., (2010). Advanced malignant melanoma responds to Prunus mume Sieb. Et Zucc (Ume) extract: Case report and in vitro study. Experimental and Therapeutic Madicine., 1(4), 569-574.

[12] Tada KI., Kawahara KI., Matsushita S., Hashiguchi T., Maruyama I., Kanekura T., (2012). MK615, a Prunus mume Steb. Et Zucc ('Ume') extract, attenuates the growth of A375 melanoma cells by inhibiting the ERK1/2-Id-1 pathway. *Phytother Res.*, 26(6), 833-838.

[13] Sunaga N., Hiraishi K., Ishizuka T., Kaira K., Iwasaki Y., Jimma F., Adachi M., Mori M., (2012) MK615, A Compound Extract from the Japanese Apricot "Prunus mume" Inhibits In vitro Cell Growth and

Interleukin-8 Expression in Non-small Cell Lung Cancer Cells. *Journal of Cancer Science and Thera*py., S11-002 (online publication).

[14] Hokari A., Ishikawa T., Tajiri H., Matsuda T., Ishii O., Matsumoto N., Okuse C., Takahashi H., Kurihara T., Kawahara KI., Maruyama I., Zuniya M., (2012). Efficacy of MK615 for the treatment of patients with liver disorders. *World J Gastroenterol.*, 18(31), 4118-4126.

[15] Miyazawa M., Utsunomiya H., Inada K., Yamada T., Okuno Y., Tatematsu M., (2006). Inhibition of Helicobacter pylori Motility by (+)-Syringaresinol from Unripe Japanese Apricot. *Biol Pharm Bull.*, 29, 172-173.

[16] Enomoto S., Yanaoka K., Utsunomiya H., Niwa T., Inada K., Ichinose M., (2010). Inhibitory effects of Japanese apricot (Prunus mume Siebold et Zucc.; Ume) on Helicobacter pylori-related chronic gastritis. *Eur J Clin Nutr.*, 64, 714-719.

[17] Otsuka T., Tsukamoto T., Tanaka H., Inada K., Utsunomiya H., Mizoshita T., Kumagai T., Katsuyama T., Miki K., Tatematsu M., (2005). Suppressive effects of fruit-juice concentrate of Prunus mume Sieb. et Zucc. (Japanese apricot, Ume) on Helicobacter pylori-induced glandular stomach lesions in Mongolian gerbils. *Asian. Pac. J. Cancer. Prev.,* 6(3), 337-341.

[18] Nakajima S., Fujita K., Inoue Y., Nishino M., Seto Y., (2006). Effect of the folk remedy, Bainiku-ekisu, a concentrate of Prunus mume juice, on Helicobacter pylori infection in humans. *Helicobacter.*, 11(6), 589-591.

[19] Lu J., Kobayashi R., Brill SJ., (1996). Characterization of a high mobility group 1/2 homolog in yeast. *J. Biol. Chem.*, 271, 33678-33685.

[20] Wang H., Bloom O., Zhang M., Vishnubhakat JM., Ombrellino M., Che J., Frazier A., Yang H., Ivanova S., Borovikova L., Manogue KR., Faist E., Abraham E., Andersson J., Andersson U., Molina PE., Abumrad NN., Sama A., Tracey KJ., (1999). HMG-1 as a late mediator of endotoxin lethality in mice. *Science.,* 285, 248-251.

[21] Taniguchi N., Kawahara K., Yone K., Hashiguchi T., Yamakuchi M., Goto M., Inoue K., Yamada S., Ijiri K., Matsunaga S., Nakajima T., Komiya S., Maruyama I., (2003). High mobility group box chromosomal protein 1 plays a role in the pathogenesis of rheumatoid arthritis as a novel cytokine. *Arthritis. Rheum.*, 48, 971-981.

[22] Kawahara K., Biswas KK., Unoshima M., Ito T., Kikuchi K., Morimoto Y., Iwata M., Tancharoen S., Oyama Y., Takenouchi K., Nawa Y., Arimura N., Jie MX., Shrestha B., Miura N., Shimizu T., Mera K., Arimura S., Taniguchi N., Iwasaka H., Takao S., Hashiguchi T.,

Maruyama I., (2008). C-reactive protein induces high mobility group box-1 protein release through a p38MAPK in the macrophage cell line RAW264.7 cells. *Cardiovasc. Pathol.*, 17, 129-138.

[23] Morimoto Y., Kawahara KI., Tancharoen S., Kikuchi K., Matsuyama T., Hashiguchi T., Izumi Y., Maruyama I., (2008). Tumor necrosis factor-alpha stimulates gingival epithelial cells to release high mobility-group box 1. J. *Periodontal. Res.*, 43, 76-83.

[24] Ito T., Kawahara K., Nakamura T., Yamada S., Nakamura T., Abeyama K., Hashiguchi T., Maruyama I., (2007). High-mobility group box 1 protein promotes development of microvascular thrombosis in rats. *J. Thromb. Haemost.,* 5, 109-116.

[25] Porto A., Palumbo R., Pieroni M., Aprigliano G., Chiesa R., Sanvito F., Maseri A., Bianchi ME., (2006). Smooth muscle cells in human atherosclerotic plaques secrete and proliferate in response to high mobility group box 1 protein. *FASEB J.*, 20, 2565-2566.

[26] Papapanou P. N., (1996). Periodontal diseases: *Epidemiology. Ann. Periodontal.,* 1 (1), 1-36.

[27] Loe H., Theilade E., Jensen S. B. (1965). Experimental gingivitis in man. *J. Periodontol.*, 36, 177-187.

[28] Slots J., Listgarten MA., (1988). *Bacteroides gingivalis*, *Bacteroides intermedius and Actinobacillus actinomycetemcomitans* in human periodontal diseases. *J. Clin. Periodontol.*, 15, 85–93.

[29] Genco CA., Van Dyke T., Amar S., (1998). Animal models for *Porphyromonas gingivalis*-mediated periodontal disease. *Trends. Microbiol.*, 6, 444-449.

[30] Holt SC., Ebersole. J, Felton J., Brunsvold M., Kornman KS., (1988). Implantation of *Bacteroides gingivalis* in nonhuman primates initiates progress of periodontitis. *Science.,* 239, 55-57.

[31] Henderson B., Poole S., Wilson M., (1996). Bacterial modulins: a novel class of virulence factors which cause host tissue pathology by inducing cytokine synthesis. *Microbiol. Rev.*, 60, 316–341.

[32] Birkedal-Hansen H., (1993). Role of cytokines and inflammatory mediators in tissue destruction. *J. Periodont. Res.,* 28, 500–510.

[33] Okada H., Murakami S., (1998). Cytokine expression in periodontal health and disease. *Crit. Rev. Oral. Biol. Med.*, 9, 248–266.

[34] Bodet C., Chandad F., Grenier D., (2006). Anti-inflammatory activity of a high-molecular-weight cranberry fraction on macrophages stimulated by lipopolysaccharides from periodontopathogens. *J. Dent. Res.*, 85, 235–239.

[35] Kim J., Amar S., (2006). Periodontal disease and systemic conditions: a bidirectional relationship. *Odontology.,* 94, 10-21.

[36] Petersen PE., (2003). The World Oral Health Report 2003: Continuous improvement of oral health in the 21st century- -the approach of the WHO Global Oral Health Programme. *Community Dent Oral Epidemiol.*, 31, 3–23.

[37] Freedman ML., Tanzer JM., (1974). Dissociation of plaque formation from glucan induced agglutination in mutants of Streptococcus mutans. *Infect Immun.*, 10, 189-196.

[38] Tanzer JM., Freedman ML., Fitzgerald RJ., Larson RH., (1974). Diminished virulence of glucan synthesis defective mutants of Streptococcus mutans. *Infect Immun.*, 10, 197-203.

[39] Murata RM., Branco de Almeida LS., Yatsuda R., Dos Santos MH., Nagem TJ., Koo H., (2008). Inhibitory effects of 7-epiclusianone on glucan synthesis, acidogenicity and biofilm formation by Streptococcus mutans. *FEMS Microbiol Lett.*, 282, 174-181.

[40] Edwardsson S., (1968). Characteristics of caries-inducing human streptococci resembling Streptococcus mutans. *Arch Oral Biol.,* 13, 637-646.

[41] Hamilton-Miller JM., (2001). Anti-cariogenic properties of tea (Camellia sinensis). *J Med Microbiol.*, 50, 299-302.

[42] Ooshima T., Osaka Y., Sasaki H., Osawa K., Yasuda H., Matsumura M., (2000). Caries inhibitory activity of cacao bean husk extract in in-vitro and animal experiments. *Arch Oral Biol.*, 45, 639-645.

[43] Makimura M., Hirasawa M., Kobayashi K., Indo J., Sakanaka S., Taguchi T., Otake S., (1993). Inhibitory effect of tea catechins on collagenase activity. *J. Periodontol.,* 64, 630-636.

[44] Bodet C., La VD., Epifano F., Grenier D., (2008). Naringenin has anti-inflammatory properties in macrophage and ex vivo human whole-blood models. *J. Periodontal. Res.*, 43, 400-407.

[45] Bodet C., Grenier D., Chandad F., Ofek I., Steinberg D., Weiss EI., (2008). Potential oral health benefits of cranberry. *Crit. Rev. Food. Sci.* Nutr., 48, 672-680.

[46] Paquette DW., Williams RC., (2000). Modulation of host inflammatory mediators as a treatment strategy for periodontal diseases. *Periodontol.* 2000., 24, 239-252.

[47] Morimoto Y., Kawahara KI., Kikuchi K., Ito T., Tokuda M., Matsuyama T., Noma S., Hashiguchi T., Torii M., Maruyama I., (2009). MK615 attenuates Porphyromonas gingivalis lipopolysaccharide-induced pro-

inflammatory cytokine release via MAPK inactivation in murine macrophage-like RAW264.7 cell. *Biochemical and Biophysical Research Communications.*, 389, 90-94.

[48] Morimoto-Yamashita Y., Kawakami Y., Tatsuyama S., Miyashita K., Emoto M., Kikuchi K., Kawahara KI., Tokuda M., (2015). A natural therapeutic approach for the treatment of periodontitis by MK615. *Med Hypotheses., in press.*

[49] Matsuzaki H., Kobayashi H., Yagyu T., (2004). Bikunin inhibits lipopolysaccharide- induced tumor necrosis factor-alpha induction in macrophages. *Clin. Diag. Lab. Immunol.*, 11, 1140–1147.

[50] Kim Do Y., Jun JH., Lee HL., Woo KM., Ryoo HM., Kim GS., Baek JH., Han SB., (2007). N-acetylcysteine prevents LPS-induced pro-inflammatory cytokines and MMP2 production in gingival fibroblasts. *Arch. Pharm. Res.*, 30, 1283-1292.

[51] Son YH., Jeong YT., Lee KA., Choi KH., Kim SM., Rhim BY., Kim K., (2008). Roles of MAPK and NF-kappaB in interleukin-6 induction by lipopolysaccharide in vascular smooth muscle cells. *J. Cardiovasc. Pharmacol.,* 51, 71-77.

[52] Neuder LE., Keener JM., Eckert RE., Trujillo JC., Jones SL., (2009). Role of p38 MAPK in LPS induced pro-inflammatory cytokine and chemokine gene expression in equine leukocytes. *Vet. Immunol. Immunopathol.,* 129: 192-199.

[53] Xiao ZY., Zhou WX., Zhang YX., Cheng JP., He JF., Yang RF., Yun LH., (2007). Inhibitory effect of linomide on lipopolysaccharide-induced proinflammatory cytokine tumor necrosis factor-alpha production in RAW264.7 macrophages through suppression of NF-κB, p38, and JNK activation. *Immunol. Lett.,* 114, 81-85.

[54] D'Acquisto F., Cicatiello L., Iuvone T., Ialenti A., Ianaro A., Esumi H., Weisz A., Carnuccio R., (1997). Inhibition of inducible nitric oxide synthase gene expression by glucocorticoid-induced protein(s) in lipopolysaccharide-stimulated J774 cells. *Eur. J. Pharmacol.*, 339, 87–95.

[55] Freedman ML., Tanzer JM., (1974). Dissociation of plaque formation from glucan induced agglutination in mutants of Streptococcus mutans. *Infect Immun.,* 10, 189-196.

[56] Tanzer JM., Freedman ML., Fitzgerald RJ., Larson RH., (1974). Diminished virulence of glucan synthesis defective *mutants* of *Streptococcus mutans*. *Infect Immun*., 10, 197-203.

[57] Makimura M., Hirasawa M., Kobayashi K., Indo J., Sakanaka S., Taguchi T., Otake S., (1993). Inhibitory effect of tea catechins on collagenase activity. *J. Periodontol.*, 64, 630-636.
[58] Morimoto-Yamashita Y., Matsuo M., Komatsuzawa H., Kawahara KI., Kikuchi K., Torii M., Tokuda M., (2011). MK615: A new therapeutic approach for the treatment of oral disease. *Medical Hypotheses.*, 77, 258-260.
[59] Wei G., Campagna NA., Bobek AL., (2006). Effect of MUC7 peptides on the growth of bacteria and on Streptococcus mutans biofilm. *J. Antimicrob. Chemother.,* 57, 1100-1009.
[60] Kozai K., Suzuki J., Okada M., Nagasaka N., (1999). Effect of oleanolic acid-cyclodextrin inclusion compounds on dental caries by in vitro experiment and rat-caries model. *Microbios.,* 97, 179-188.
[61] Kozai K., Miyake Y., Kohda H., Kametaka S., Yamasaki K., Nagasaka N., (1987) Inhibition of Glucosyltransferase from Streptococcus mutans by Oleanolic acid and Ursolic *Acid. Caries. Res.*, 21, 104-108.

In: Apricots and Peaches
Editor: Jeanne Hansen

ISBN: 978-1-63484-684-4

Chapter 3

PEACHES AND NECTARINES: PROPERTIES, DEFICIT IRRIGATION STRATEGIES AND POSTHARVEST MANAGEMENT

Natalia Falagán*[*], *Francisco Artés Calero* *and Encarna Aguayo

Postharvest and Refrigeration Group and Institute of Plant Biotechnology
Regional Campus of International Excellence 'Campus Mare Nostrum'
- Universidad Politécnica de Cartagena (UPCT). Paseo Alfonso XIII,
Cartagena, Murcia, Spain

ABSTRACT

Nowadays, Spain is the fourth largest producer of nectarine and peach with an average annual volume of 1,219,780.50 tonnes. This quantity has increased in recent years due to the new varieties obtained which are adapted to each geographical area and specific soil conditions. Also, it is due to advances in irrigation and fertilization strategies, as well as improvements in postharvest techniques and traceability that promote export opportunities. Stone fruit crops require an average of 5,000 to 7,000 m^3 of irrigation water per hectare and year. In Mediterranean areas or the southern of the United States, great nectarine and peach producers, agriculture is limited by scarce water supplies and their poor quality. Therefore, the application of irrigation strategies to optimize water use,

[*] Corresponding author: E-mail address: natalia.falagan@upct.es natalia.falagan@gmail.com.

but maintain yield and quality is essential. These techniques are generally known as regulated deficit irrigation (RDI). Their use assumes knowledge of each crop phenological stage in order to avoid possible adverse effects on both plant growth and fruit. In recent years, consumers have increasingly requested products with high sensory, microbiological and nutritional quality. Consumers are also interested in purchasing products grown under sustainable techniques. Currently, there is also an increasing interest in the consumption of fruits and vegetables with high antioxidant potential. That is to say, commodities that contain health-promoting compounds, such as vitamin C and certain individual polyphenols. Previous studies have observed an increase in these biocompounds when the product has been subjected to RDI. This is caused by the activation of specific metabolic pathways that lead to the synthesis of these biocompounds as a response to water stress. In this chapter, the production and characteristics of peaches and nectarines are contextualized. Here, the main effects of deficit irrigation on fruit quality and bioactive compounds during peach and nectarine growth and postharvest period have been taken into account. Postharvest management of these commodities either as whole product or minimally processed is explained, listing the main recommendations.

1. Introduction: Peaches and Nectarines

1.1. Origin and Characteristics

Peach trees (*Prunus persica* L. Batsch) belong to the *Rosaceae* family, *Prunoideae* subfamily, *Prunus* genus, *Amygdalus* subgenus and *persica* specie. Their origin is located in China (Thacker 1985). They have been cultivated since the early days of Chinese culture, around 2000 BC (Singh et al. 2007; Geissler 2009). Through different trade routes, peaches arrived to Persia (nowadays, Iran) from where they spread throughout the world, especially in warm climates. This subgender has three different forms: *vulgaris* or common peach, *laevis* or nectarine and *platycarpa* or flat peach. In this sense, peaches and nectarines belong to the same species, even though they are marketed as different fruits.

Both of them are classified as 'stone fruit' due to their seed, which is enclosed in a hard, stone-like endocarp. Commercially they are distinguished as 'clingstone' (pit adheres to flesh) or 'freestone' with the pit relatively free of the flesh (Siddiq et al. 2012). It is a very appropriate species for warm climates. Like other temperate fruits, peach has chilling and heat requirements for flowering. Its blooming date depends on these 'chilling requirements,' varying between 50 and 1,500 hours under 7ºC depending on the cultivar (cv.) according to Bassiand Monet (2008). The main difference between peaches and nectarines is that nectarines are smooth-skinned fuzzless while peaches are characterized by a fuzzy skin. The lack of fuzz is due to a single gene (Anon, 2008).

Peaches and nectarines share the same phenology. The term phenology refers to the annual calendar of plant biological events. It includes phases such as budburst and swelling, shoot growth and increments in trunk diameter and root dynamics as well as reproductive growth (flower initiation, fruit setting, and fruit maturing) according to Mounzer et al. (2008). Growers need to know and understand the growth stages of all agricultural crops to design irrigation and fertilization programs. Bleiholder et al. (1989) defined a scale, called BBCH, which describes the phenological stages of both herbaceous and woody plants (Mounzer et al. 2008). Besides these identifiers, three stages have been determined in peach and nectarine fruit growth (Figure 2). Its development is characterized by a double sigmoid curve pattern (Connors 1919). In the first stage, cell division occurs (I), then a slow growth phase (II) and finally, the third stage showing cell expansion (III), with rapid fruit growth until reaching their final size (Figure 2).

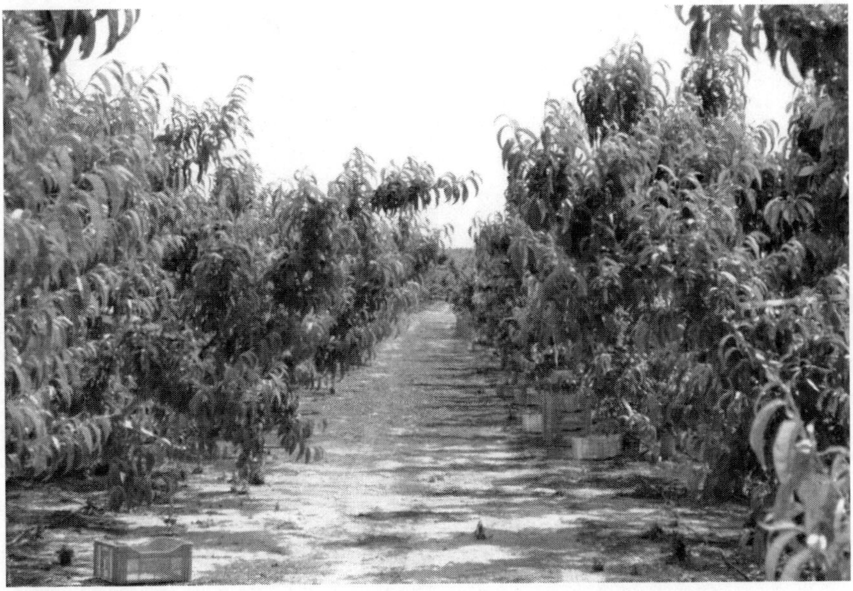

Figure 1. Nectarine field during harvest period.

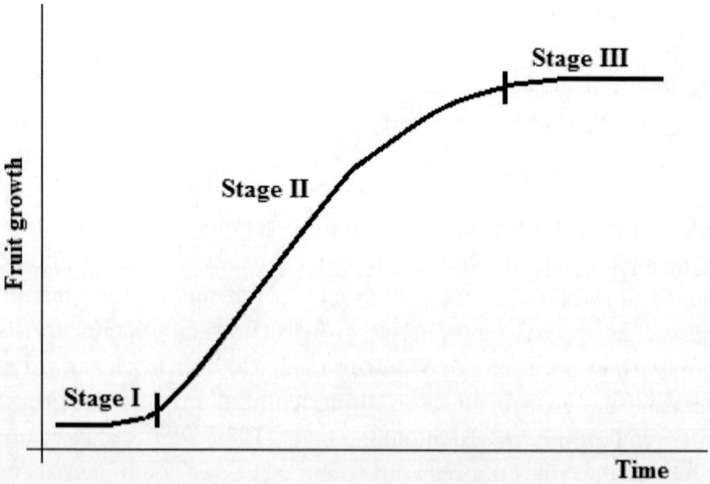

Figure 2. Different stages of fruit growth in stone fruit.

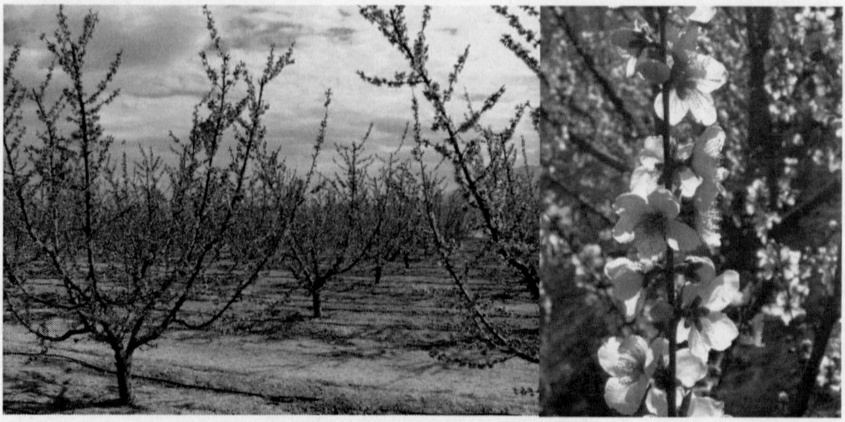

Figure 3. Flowering phenological state in peach fruit.

In this sense, in stone fruit trees, the critical periods for irrigation mainly occur during the second stage of rapid growth of the fruit and during the flower induction/differentiation (Ruiz-Sánchez et al. 1999; Torrecillas et al. 2000). In the first case, the fruit size is affected and the total soluble solids content (SSC) increases (Torrecillas et al. 2000; Naor 2001), while the water deficit during flower induction/differentiation, that occurs after harvesting, is very critical because it can affect the yield of the following year (Ruiz-Sánchez et al. 1999; Torrecillas et al. 2000). Nevertheless, if an excessive deficit is avoided in that phenological moment, some preliminary results mention how to induce an improvement of fruit quality in the following harvest (Gelly et al. 2004; Dichio et al. 2004; Dichio et al. 2007).

1.2. Economic Importance and World Distribution

World production of peaches and nectarines is led by China with around 60% of world production, followed by Europe with a 23.5% worldwide production (Figure 4 and 5). Spain is the fourth producer country with an average production of 1,219,780 t in the period 2000-2013 (FAOSTAT 2015), as observed in Figure 4. In fact, peach is nowadays the main deciduous fruit species produced in Spain with a surface of 76,000 ha in 2010 (MAGRAMA 2015). The observed increasing trend with time is due to the improvement of technology of production, which includes new cvs. and rootstocks, training systems, fertilization or pest and disease management (Iglesias 2013).

Spain has introduced in the last decade a great number of new cvs. covering a wide range of maturity, with different size, appearance and fruit taste (Iglesias et al. 2005; 2007; 2010b).

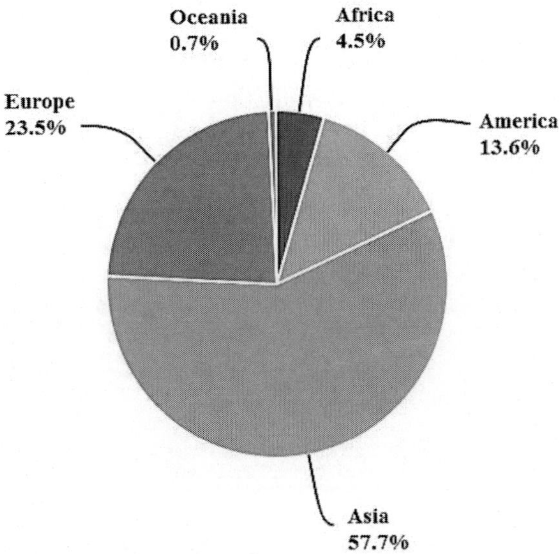

Figure 4. Average peach and nectarine production share by region in the period 2000-2013. FAOSTAT 2015.

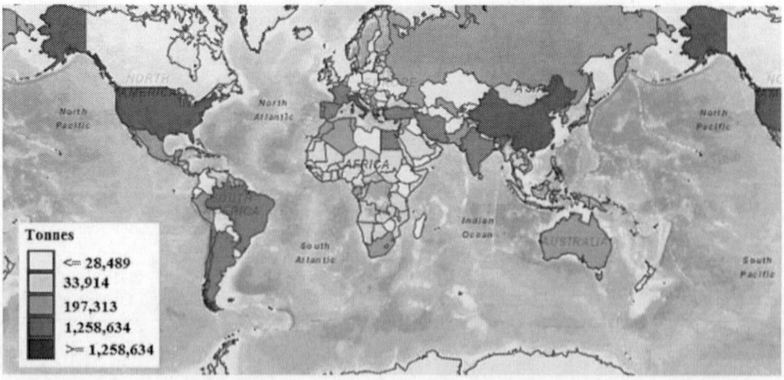

Figure 5. Average peach and nectarine worldwide production in the period 2000-2013. FAOSTAT 2015.

New specific rootstocks adapted in a great diversity of soil conditions (Moreno 2005; Jiménez et al. 2011) make possible the increase of cropped surface.

Besides the above mentioned advances in irrigation, fertilization, crop protection, postharvest technology, certification and traceability, allowed in the last two decades a consistent improvement of the competitiveness of Spain, in particular to export markets (Iglesias2010a) mainly of European countries (Figure 6).

In Spain, the Region of Murcia is the third producer, behind Aragon and Catalonia. The surface cultivated with this crop in the Region of Murcia represents nearly 22.5% of the total surface cultivated in Spain. This proportion is increasing year by year.

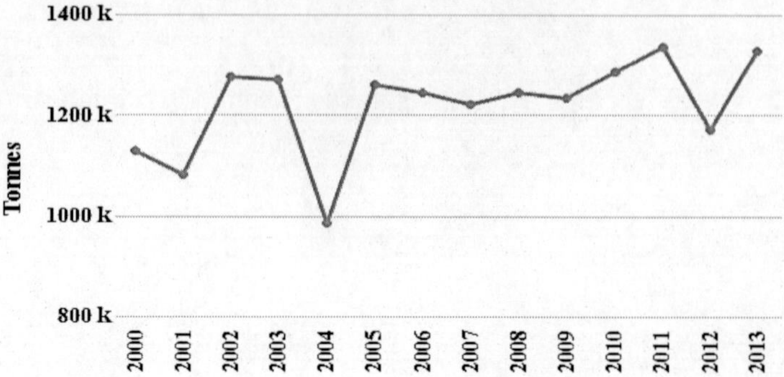

Figure 6. Average peach and nectarine Spanish production in the period 2000-2013. FAOSTAT 2015.

1.3. Produce Facts and Consumption

In general, stone fruits are nutritionally important because consumer acceptance is very high, being one of the most significant fruits during spring and summer. However, their total antioxidant potential is lower that other fruits such as strawberry, kiwifruit, apple and orange. Their main source of antioxidant compounds are phenolics and also vitamin C and carotenoids. The following Table 1 lists the nutrition information of peaches and nectarines. It is important to highlight the mineral content available in these stone fruits.

These commodities are destined for the fresh market, but both of them are also used in processing. Depending on the peach or nectarine type, the fruit have different destinations. Freestone peaches and nectarines are more commonly destined for the fresh market while clingstone ones are mostly used in processing. This is due to the difficulty in separating the flesh from the stone in clingstone varieties, so it is more convenient to use freestone cvs. For fresh-cut (FC) produce.

Peaches and nectarines can be consumed fresh, or added to salads and smoothies. Nowadays they are also used as a topping for yogurt or ice cream. If they are dried peaches and nectarines are a great supplement in cereals. Other options include freezing, canning or serving as nectar or jam.

Table 1. Nutrition Information for Raw Fruits (peaches). U.S. Food and Drug Administration (Double serving = DV)

Fruits Serving Size (gram weight)	Peach medium (147 g)
Calories	60
Calories from Fat	0
Total Fat (g)	0.5
Sodium (mg)	0
Potassium (mg)	230
Total Carb. (g)	15
Dietary Fiber (g)	2
Sugars (g)	13
Protein (g)	1
Vitamin A (%DV)	6
Vitamin C (%DV)	15
Calcium (%DV)	0
Iron (%DV)	2

1.4. Disorders

Peaches and nectarines suffer postharvest deterioration, with mechanical injuries and temperature being the main causes. In the following lines, some of the most important disorders are listed.

a) Physiological Disorders and Physical Damages

Internal Breakdown or Chilling Injury (CI). Usually, ripe stone fruits decay quickly at room temperature. Hence, cold storage is used to slow down deterioration processes. In this case, the pathology develops faster and more intensely when susceptible fruit are stored at temperatures between 2.2 and 7.6°C (killing temperature zone) than those stored at 0°C or below but above their freezing point (Harding and Haller, 1934, Crisosto et al. 1999; Luchsinger and Artés 2000; Lurie and Crisosto 2005). These symptoms are detected when fruit reaches consumers (Bruhn et al. 1991; Crisosto et al. 1995). Visually, they develop after 1-2 weeks when fruit are stored at 2–5°C. Genetic factors also influence the impact of CI on stone fruit development. Recently, Puig et al. (2015) reported that in sensitive fruit a cold response program is activated and regulated by auxin distribution and ethylene and these hormones have a role in sensitivity to CI even before fruit are cold stored. CI manifests itself as dry, mealy, woolly (lack of juice; Figure 7) or hard textured fruit with no juice (leatheriness), flesh or pit cavity browning, and flesh bleeding or internal reddening (Fernández-Trujillo et al. 1998; Luchsinger and Artés 2000; Lurie and Crisosto 2005). When the damage advances, CI fruit also show flesh tissue separation and cavity formation. In general, nectarines are less susceptible to CI than peaches (Retamales et al. 1992; Lurie and Crisosto 2005; Crisosto 2006).

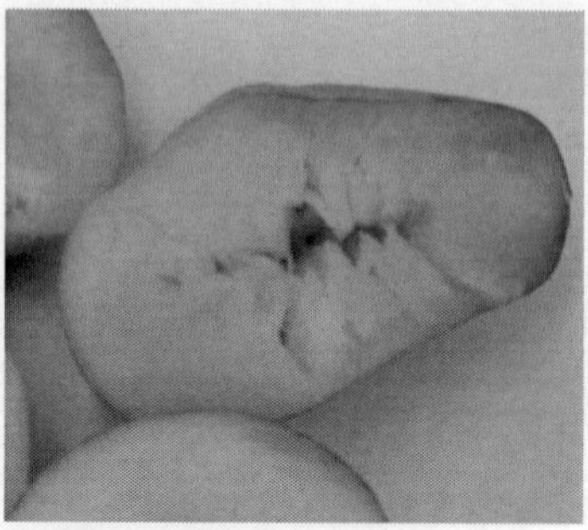

Figure 7. Wooliness in 'Flordastar' peach.

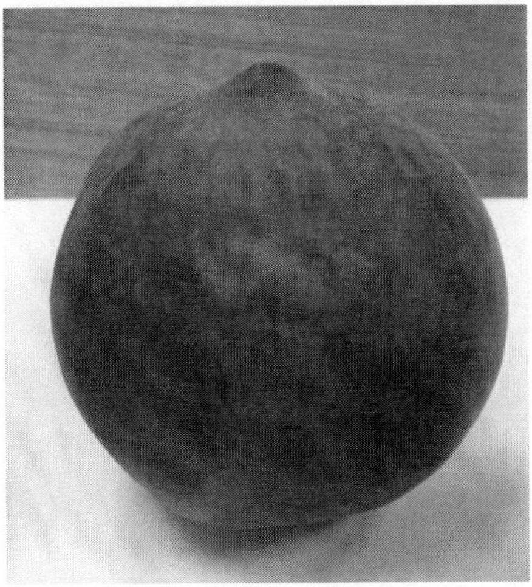

Figure 8. Inking in 'Ruby Rich' peach.

Inking. This is a cosmetic problem which affects the skin of peaches and nectarines. It can be identified visually by black or brown spots or stripes that appear 24-48 hours after harvest (Cheng and Crisosto 1994, Figure 8). It is provoked by the combination of abrasion damage and heavy metals such as iron, copper and aluminum. The abrasion damage normally occurs during harvesting and handling operations during postharvest. Inking causes important losses to the stone fruit industry every year.

b) Pathological Disorders

Brown Rot. This disease is caused by *Monilia fructicola* and is one of the most destructive disorders in stone fruits. The fungus not only affects the product but also blossoms and shoots. The infection appears during flowering and fruit rot may occur either before harvest or during postharvest.

Gray Mold. This is caused by *Boyrytis cinerea,* especially during wet spring weather. If the fruit is contaminated due to harvest and handling damage, the first symptoms will appear during storage. To prevent this, it is important to avoid mechanical injuries and control temperature and relative humidity during postharvest.

Rhizopus Rot. As its name implies, this is mainly caused by *Rhizopus stolonifera*. Normally, the first signs occur in ripened fruit kept at 20 to 25°C. Respecting the recommended storage temperature (always under 5ºC) should be enough to control this fungal attack (Figure 9).

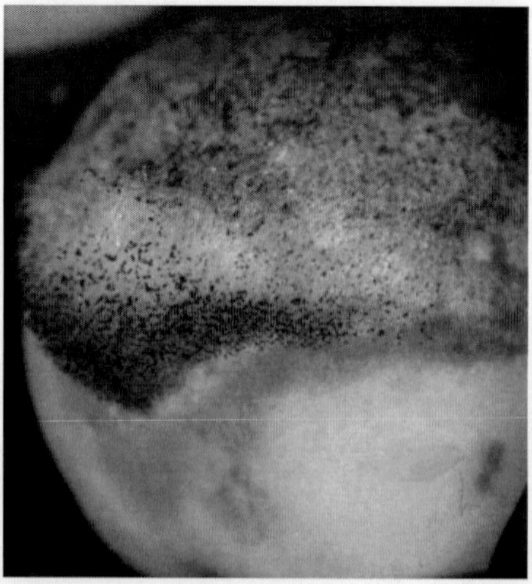

Figure 9. *Rhizopus nigricans* in 'Sudanell' peach.

1.5. Importance of Extra Early Cultivars

Stone fruit trees present a low spontaneous mutational rate from an agronomical viewpoint. Breeding programs have some difficulties in the development of new cvs. due to the breeding cycles, heterozygosity, polyploidy, and long field evaluation procedures (Tiang et al. 2009). Nowadays, around 70 breeding programs in the world work on finding cvs. able to adapt to a variety of cultivation conditions.

One of the objectives of the breeding programs is to obtain peach and nectarine trees with early blooming (Carusso and Sottile 1999; George and Nissen 1992). The final aim consists of the spreading of the harvest period to cover the peach and nectarine market throughout the year (Carusso and Sottile 1999; Byrne2003; Badenes et al. 2006; Martínez-Calvo et al. 2006). Peach and nectarine are mainly sent to the European markets and they maintain their economic significance and their competitiveness in the sector thanks to the relatively high prices reached due to early production (Alvisi et al. 1995). However, due to their characteristics, their cultivation requires areas with high temperatures and short winters, as found in Mediterranean areas, which face intense periods of drought. Despite this, the irrigation management of these crops implies high water amounts (5,000-7,000 m^3 ha^{-1} $year^{-1}$).

In general, peach and nectarine trees are highly sensitive to drought stress at particular phenological stages, such as flowering and fruiting, and during stem extension and fruit growth (Berman and DeJong 1997; Xiloyannis et al. 2005; Dichio et al. 2007). These periods are considered to be 'critical.' During them, their water demand should be met for a better working of the plant system. However, there are few references to early ripening cvs., whereas important physiological changes have been reported among peach cvs.in relation to their maturation date (Mercier et al. 2009).

In this work, two extra early cvs. have been selected (Figure 10):

- Peach **'Flordastar'**: among the extra early cvs. of peach, 'Flordastar' must be highlighted due to the good adaptation to warm areas without frost risk. This genotype has been obtained in Florida University (Gainesville. USA). It is also known as 'Sherman.' The tree is semi-erect, being a vigorous cv. Their flowers are pink and their fructification occurs in mixed stems and it is very intense. Its productivity is high. Blooming period: last week of January. Maturation period: second week of May. The peach is round, 70-80% red color over yellow ground. The firmness level is medium and the general caliber is A-B category. Among extra early cvs., this one is the least exigent in chilling requirements.
- Nectarine **'VioWhite 5'**: this genotype has been obtained by natural crossings Planasa in Cartaya, Huelva (Spain). It is a cv. protected with the register number: EU 1667 (23-10-01). The tree is semi-erect, being a vigorous cv. Their flowers are pink and their fructification occurs in mixed stems and it is very intense. Blooming period: last week of January. Maturation period: last week of April. It is a round nectarine, with red skin and white pulp. It is the earliest cv.in the market.

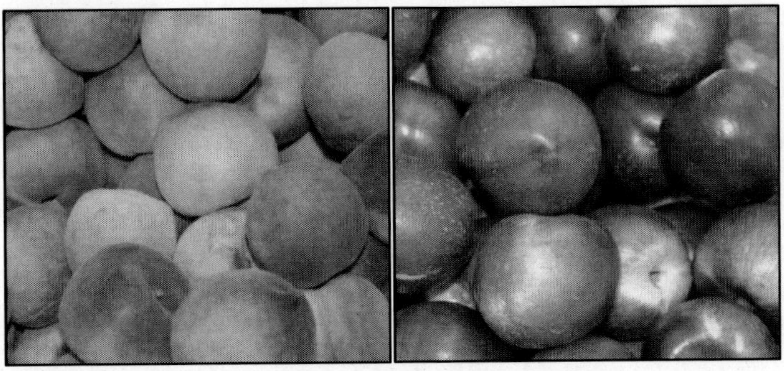

Figure 10. 'Flordastar' peach and 'VioWhite 5' nectarine.

For these cvs., about 75% of seasonal evapotranspiration (ET) occurs after harvest (Johnson et al. 1992). It means that its high water necessities match with low evaporative demand periods (Falagán et al. 2014). Definitively, the interest in extra early cvs. lies in the fact that their maximum irrigation needs are in periods of relatively low evaporative demand, they can introduce fruits in the market in periods of low stone fruit competition, and that they are low cold-hours demanding, so they can be considered as an alternative in most agricultural areas of the Mediterranean basin.

1.6. Quality Concept and Characteristics

Quality concept has been defined as the physico-chemical characteristics, which offer the consumer a commodity with good appearance and high acceptance level (Kramer and Twigg 1966). This concept involves the combination of characteristics that determines the value of produce to the consumers, who expect a product without defects, in optimum maturity and in fresh condition. To achieve this good acceptance, quality indexes at harvest should be taken into account. The most common quality indexes to determine harvest date in peaches and nectarines are caliber, titratable acidity (TA), soluble solid content (SSC), pulp firmness and skin color.

In order to obtain TA, the titration method is used. This is a chemical process used in establishing the amount of constituent substance in a sample, in this case acids, by using a standard reagent such as NaOH. In this sense, classification in different categories is useful to evaluate quality. Iglesias and Echeverría (2009) reported an acidity scale as follows: subacid cvs. (0-4 g malic acid L^{-1}), sweet (4-9 g malic acid L^{-1}), equilibrated (9-15 g malic acid L^{-1}) and finally acid cvs. (> 15 g malic acid L^{-1}).

SSC is one of the main quality parameters used in food and beverage analysis. It is defined as those substances which can be part of a solution such as sugars and salts. Several studies on peaches and nectarines have related the higher consumer acceptance with a higher concentration in SSC (Mitchell et al. 1990; Parker et al. 1991). In fact, some new early cvs. can reach 13 ºBrix. Hilaire and Mathieu (2004) reported that values of acceptance over 70% are reached when peaches and nectarines contained a minimum of 10 ºBrix. They also stated that a satisfactory firmness should be under 49 N. Firmness not only is a good quality index but also can indicate shelf-life potential in peaches and nectarines. Firmness values offer maturity stage information and its harvest level should be maintained at the moment of consumption. According to Crisosto et al. (2001), fruits under 27 N are susceptible to mechanical damage during postharvest handling. In this sense, peaches and nectarines have been classified as 'ready to buy' (26.5-35.3 N) and 'ready to eat'(9-13.5 N) (Crisosto and Labavitch 2002). Temperature is the key factor that affects the evolution of firmness, with the pectin esterase and polygalacturonase cell wall degrading enzymes playing an essential role in peaches and nectarines (Salmerón and Artés 1991; Artés et al. 1996).

Skin color is one of the parameters that consumers use to identify maturity stage (Wills et al. 2007). It is known that color is the result of biochemical changes, such as chlorophyll degradation through chlorophyllase (EC 3.1.1.14) an intrinsic membrane-bound enzyme located in photosynthetic membrane systems, together with other related chlorophyll catabolism enzymes (Dangl et al. 2000; Artés et al. 2002). Either in peaches or nectarines, chlorophyll concentration tends to decrease with ripening, increasing other compounds such as carotenoids, flavonoids or anthocyanins. All of these are also responsible of the changes in peel and pulp color. The speed of these changes depends on cv. and environmental conditions. In general, CIELAB scale is used to monitor color, with a* values being the best parameter to indicate color changes during ripening, with their level increasing, while L*, b*, hue angle and chroma change slightly (Nunes and Emond 2002).

2. Deficit Irrigation Strategies

2.1. Concept

'Water and all that relies on it, from food to sanitation and public health, is an emblematic aspect of climate change whose urgency people tend to instantly understand,' said Hans Joachim Schellnhuber, director of the Potsdam Institute for Climate Impact Research in Germany.

Nowadays, multidisciplinary groups are working on models which have found that climate-driven changes in evaporation and precipitation will result in a 40% increase in the number of people worldwide who must make do with less than 500 m^3/year of water, which is a common threshold for 'water scarcity' (Schiermeier 2014). These modelers considered that parts of the southern United States, the Mediterranean and the Middle East were the regions most at risk from water scarcity. Besides the lack of quantity and quality of water resources in these areas, the situation is worsened by the competition for the available water with other non-agricultural uses (Conejero et al. 2011).

In this sense, under this water scarcity situation, when water is not available to fully satisfy crop irrigation requirements, new and accurate tools are needed (Pereira et al. 2012). In general, most irrigation water is obtained directly from surface or groundwater sources and applied using overhead methods (Knox et al. 2012). The quantity applied and the moment of application should fit with crop water requirements in each phenological period. In this regard, biological and physical criteria must be established to develop more precise irrigation management practices (Goldhamer and Fereres 2001; Pereira et al. 2002; Naor 2006; Katerji et al. 2008).

Currently, techniques such as regulated deficit irrigation (RDI), an irrigation strategy, which aims to save water with a minimum impact on yield and fruit quality, are being developed (Chalmers et al. 1989; Goldhamer 1989; Naor 2006). The use of RDI to schedule irrigation in orchards was considered as an efficient strategy for water saving (Mitchell and Chalmers 1982; Mitchell et al. 1989). This technique was firstly developed in Australia with the initial aim of limiting the plant growth of excessively vigorous fruit trees, especially peach and pear (Mitchell and Chalmers 1982; Mitchell et al. 1984; Mitchell et al. 1986). Its application involves accurate knowledge of crop behavior in each phenological stage, to apprehend their requirements in every phase of crop and fruit development. It is essential to identify the periods where the possible adverse effects of a deficit irrigation on plant and fruit development are minimized, considered as non-critical periods.

As mentioned above, these periods are well defined in stone fruit trees (Torrecillas et al. 2000). In these trees, there are two critical points: the first one corresponds to the second rapid fruit growth period (stage III). In this phase, a severe reduction of water supply can reduce fruit size and subsequently, productivity (Figure 2). The second critical point occurs in the early postharvest phase. In this period, a severe water stress can affect flower bud induction and/or the floral differentiation processes (Faust 1989). It can also have an effect on the carbohydrate reserve accumulation (Oliveira and Priestley 1988). Starch reserves have an important influence on the following harvest, as López et al. (2007) demonstrated on peach trees.

Currently, irrigation program planning is designed through the study of plant-based water status indicators (Shackel et al. 1997; Fernández and Cuevas 2010). Ortuño et al. (2010) remarked that plant water status regulates many physiological processes and this fact must be taken into account. One of these indicators is able to measure daily trunk diameter fluctuations with high precision and is called maximum daily trunk shrinkage (MDS) according to Huguet et al. (1990) and Ortuño et al. (2010). MDS is considered to be the most sensitive water stress indicator in peach (Goldhamer et al. 1999) and in olive (Moriana and Fereres 2002). This tool considers the daily trunk diameter fluctuations, modelling a curve of shrinkage and swelling that occurs in plants (Corell et al. 2014). These fluctuations are due to the tension created in the xylem from the evaporative surface of the leaves to every organ of the plant when transpiration begins early in the morning (Fernández and Cuevas 2010). Then, during the night, part of the water stored in the plant tissues is lost, allowing the plant to respond to changes in atmospheric demand (Hinckley and Bruckerhoff 1975). This event occurs in every water-storing organ of the plant, including the stem, branches, roots, leaves and fruits (Ueda and Shibata 2001; Sevanto et al. 2002; Čermák et al. 2007).

These changes should be recorded during the day. The first scientific systems measured stem growth using tapes or callipers, with low-precision accuracy (Marsham 1759). Then, it the late 1800s, highly sensitive dendrometers and dendrographs were developed (Figure 11). During that time, the equipment was highly complicated, so it became more popular when the technology was modernized. Nowadays, they are automated and they can measure the fluctuations with different types of dendrometers: radial (measuring growth along a single radius), diametral (two opposing radius), and circumferential (many radius of a plant conductive organ) (Fernández and Cuevas 2010). Since the 1990s, linear variable differential transformers have been widely used to schedule irrigation. These types of sensors are robust and very precise, close to ± 1 μm. Depending on the dendrometer model, screws in the tree may be necessary either to support the instrument or to act as a fixed reference against which growth is measured (Fernández and Cuevas 2010). To avoid any damage or interference in tree growth, the dendrometer is usually attached to the stem by elastic straps made of aluminum and invar (Li et al. 1989; Doltra et al. 2007). This system allows the permanent contact of the instrument with the tree, which is essential. To reinforce it, a spring or even glue can be used (Ueda and Shibata 2001).

Dendrometer installation should be preceded by a calibration with a micrometer or standardized metal plates (Intrigliolo and Castel 2004; Sevanto et al. 2005). Dentrometers should be installed on the side of stem opposite to the sun's trajectory, in order to minimize the direct heating (Fernández and Cuevas 2010), so we can obtain a reliable MDS value.

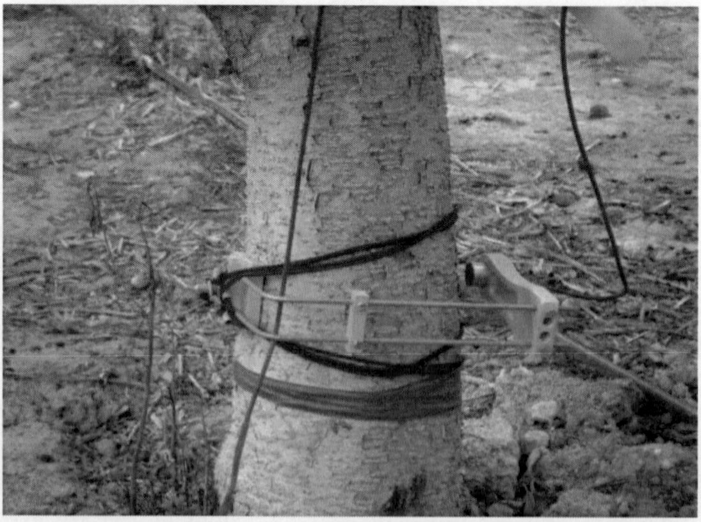

Figure 11. Dendrometer detail installed on 'VioWhite 5' nectarine tree.

From earlier studies, an increase in MDS values has been found in response to drought stress (Moriana et al. 2000; Deslauriers et al. 2003; Ortuño et al. 2006). In contrast, severe conditions of drought stress decrease MDS values (Moriana et al. 2000; Ortuño et al. 2006; Intrigliolo and Castel 2007). In this sense, the use of absolute MDS values, which do not consider the evaporative demand, is not very informative. One solution to normalize these values is the application of the concept signal intensity (SI), which considers the ratio between absolute MDS values with respect to those in non-limiting soil water conditions (actual MDS/reference MDS) (Goldhamer and Fereres 2001; Naor and Cohen 2003; Ortuño et al. 2006, 2010; De la Rosa et al. 2013).

The reference MDS values can be obtained from well-irrigated trees, considering their characteristic crop evapotranspiration coefficient or from baselines, which are calculated from reference equations and metereological data (Goldhamer and Fereres 2001). Depending on SI values, it is possible to know the stress level in the tree. SI is a dimensionless variable, in which values above unity indicate deficit irrigation, values equal to unity represent good plant water status and values below unity indicate an over irrigation situation (Conesa et al. 2014).

There are several alternatives to this method, as we will summarize in the following lines. One of them is leaf water potential. It is a direct measure of the plant water status, determined with a pressure chamber. The measurement system is based on applying pressure on the leaf blade which is placed inside the chamber except for the petiole which projects outside through an orifice. Then, the pressure is slowly increased until the onset of sap drops through the visible petiole. At this moment, the applied pressure corresponds to the leaf water potential (Turner 1981).

Another option commonly and widely used is sap flow measurement. This allows the study of tree-level water fluxes and water use of forest ecosystems (Hölttäa et al. 2015). In general, these systems are based on sensing convective heat transfer inside the tree stems and branches, through heat carried with the sap stream. This method is very sensitive and allows the calculation of the plant water requirements. The fluctuations that occur during the day permit the interpretation of the water situation at each moment.

These are some of the most used methods nowadays. Definitively, the final aim of these technologies is to obtain an optimum irrigation scheduling which provides a good water supply for productivity while adjusting to plant necessities, in order to save water resources. The choice of one of these methods depends on budget (more or less sophisticated methods are available), precision needed and time and operators involved in the measurement.

2.2. Effect of RDI Strategies on Fruit Quality

The application of RDI strategies not only has water saving benefits, but also reduces excessive vegetative growth as previously mentioned, maintaining yield. If applied with a good knowledge of critical periods it may improve fruit quality (Behboudian et al. 2011; Faci et al. 2014). Firstly, there are some studies which found that stem potentials of about -1.5 MPa provoked reductions in photosynthesis that could be compensated by the reduction in the growth rate of vegetative apexes (Shackel 2000), which are the major carbohydrate sinks during postharvest stage (Dichio et al. 2007). Thanks to this vigor regulation, the competition for assimilates between reserve tissues and vegetative apexes decreases, improving light interception and reducing summer pruning (Boland et al. 2000) with the subsequent better crop management. This event has been largely observed in peach and nectarine trees (Larson et al. 1988; Johnson et al. 1992; Ghrab et al. 1998). This advantage occurs when water stress is applied after flowering. However, if this stress is induced during flowering, RDI may inhibit fertilization, reduce fruit set and increase fruit abscission.

Secondly, marketable crop yield is closely related to the total amount of water evapotranspired (Stewart et al. 1977; Hexem and Heady 1978;

Doorenbos and Kassam 1979; Taylor et al. 1983). In this sense, it is also related to the biomass production. Some studies reported that a reduction in yield can occur due to water deficit, due to a decrease in biomass production and/or by a decrease in the fraction of biomass that is harvested (Fereres and Soriano 2007). However, not all studies report reductions. Teviotdale et al. (2001), Shackel (2002), Gelly et al. (2004) and Geerts and Raes (2009) found that mild to moderate water stress had little or no impact on yield, even increasing it (Goldhamer et al. 2006). All of these studies highlighted the importance of the moment at which RDI should be applied. Regarding size, some studies consider a diameter reduction while others reflect on the moment of application for different responses. Moderate RDI applied during cell division or rapid endocarp hardening improved fruit size (Vallverdú et al. 2012), while during main fruit-growth stage, RDI could negatively impact on this parameter (Urban et al. 2014).

Thirdly, important characteristics of fruit quality including appearance, texture or taste are influenced by environmental conditions such as irrigation (Génard et al. 2007). Improvement in fruit quality has been generally identified with an increase in SSC, which implies a better acceptance by consumers who generally prefer a sweeter fruit taste (Li et al. 1989; Crisosto et al. 1994; Ben Mechlia et al. 2002; Vallverdú et al. 2012). Taste is also related to acidity. Previous studies reported that pH and acidity were not affected by RDI (Layne and Tan 1984; Crisosto et al. 1994; Crisosto et al. 1997). These authors also remarked that no influence was found on firmness, which is determinant for consumer acceptance and impacts on organoleptic quality, shelf-life and transportability (Urban et al. 2014). Another important quality parameter is color. Chlorophylls, carotenoids and anthocyanins are the responsible for peach and nectarine fruit colour. During ripening the thylakoids are reorganised and chloroplasts containing chorophylls are gradually replaced by chromoplast containing only carotenoids. Anthocyanins are contened in vacuolar juice, mainly in mature epidermal cells, although they also accumulate in flesh tissue (Artés et al. 2002). The existence of pigments responsible for coloration such as anthocyanins, carotenoids and chlorophylls is influenced by lowered water status situations (Behboudian and Mills 1997). Some studies reported that the accumulation of sugars can play an important role in pigment development (Mills et al. 1994).

Besides these events, some authors add more benefits: reduced weight loss and fungal attacks have been also reported (Crisosto et al. 1994; Pérez-Pastor et al. 2007; Falagán et al. 2014; Mpelasoka et al. 2014). These parameters are considered important for postharvest handling and shipping of stone fruit

(Crisosto et al. 1994). The first reduction is normally attributed to the formation of a thicker cuticle provoked by water stress, which acts as water loss block. Weight loss is highly related to firmness. In general, the higher the weight loss, the lower the firmness. This is important because consumers consider firmness as one of the most important parameters in order to score quality.

2.3. Effect of RDI Strategies on Bioactive Compounds and Metabolic Activity

The high concentration and variety of secondary metabolites in plants are well known. These compounds play different roles in biological processes like resistance to biotic and abiotic stresses. In general, compounds derived from secondary metabolism have been associated with interaction between plants and environmental factors such as: herbivores, insects, pathogens, pollinators, etc. These substances are essential in growth and development of plants and fruit, as well as resistance to abiotic stresses such as water stress.

The consumption of fruit supplies a wide range of health-promoting phytochemicals (or bioactive compounds). These compounds are mainly represented by vitamin C and polyphenols such as anthocyanins, phenolic acids, flavanols and (Urban et al. 2014), with compounds having antioxidant properties (Szajdek and Borowska 2008). Their main concentration is found in peel rather than in pulp. This is why it is important for the consumer to consider peel as an edible part and avoid casting it aside. The reason why they are considered to be antioxidants is due to the ability of scavenging reactive oxygen species (ROS), such as hydroxyl, peroxide radicals and radicals of other reactive forms of oxygen, including hydrogen peroxide and singlet oxygen. Besides this, these compounds are able to inhibit the activity of enzymes and form complexes with metals, which catalyze oxidative reactions (Rice-Evans et al. 1995; Harborne and Williams 2000; Heim et al. 2002). Phenolic compounds are influenced by many factors, such as the cultivation, region, weather conditions, ripeness, harvesting time, storage time and conditions (Haffner et al. 2002; Anttonen and Karjalainen 2005; Ehala et al. 2005; Castrejón et al. 2008). One of their functions is to protect the plant against adverse factors such as drought, UV radiation, infections or physical damage (Benvenuti et al. 2004).

Vitamin C is one important water-soluble vitamin. Humans cannot synthesize it due to the absence of the enzyme L-gulonolactone oxidase.

Nevertheless, most plants and animals are able to synthesize it from D-glucose or D-galactose (Szajdek and Borowska 2008). Vitamin C refers to all compounds exhibiting equivalent biological activity to L-ascorbic acid (L-AsA), including its oxidation products (dehydroascorbic acid, DHA) or isomers such as isoascorbic acid (Spínola et al. 2014). As previously mentioned, L-AsA is naturally present in most fruits and vegetables. Equally, it is important to measure L-AsA and DHA, as both of them exhibit biological activity, and contribute to the total vitamin C. The oxidation of L-AsA into DHA is influenced by exposure to high temperatures and pH, light, presence of O_2 or metals (Fe^{3+}, Ag^{+}, Cu^{2+}), and through enzymatic action (Spínola et al. 2014). The proportions of L-AsA and DHA depend on pre-harvest (origin, cultivation practices, irrigation and maturity stage) and postharvest conditions (handling and storage). In fact, we have found how control samples (well irrigated) showed higher AsA concentration while showing the lowest DHA values. Meanwhile, fruits subjected to RDI treatments revealed the opposite behavior. This was because abiotic stress can influence the oxidation of AsA into DHA, through the activation of ascorbate peroxidase enzyme (Falagán et al. 2015b). In this sense, DHA levels were good indicators for the plant water status.

Environmental factors play a stimulating role in the synthesis and the accumulation of these bioactive compounds in fruits. Concretely, moderate stress and more specifically, controlled drought, appears to be a promising technique (Poiroux-Gonord et al. 2010). It has been reported that water deficit provokes an abiotic stress in the plant, promoting the concentration of bioactive compounds due to the increase of the activities of some antioxidant enzymes such as ascorbate peroxidase (APX; EC 1.11.1.11), catalase (CAT; EC 1.11.1.6) and superoxide dismutase (EC 1.15.1.1) according to Barbagallo et al. (2013) and Laribi et al. (2013). In this sense there are some studies which link this accumulation of compounds to oxidative stress that influences directly or indirectly the biosynthetic pathway of these compounds (Urban et al. 2014). Definitively, water stress can exacerbate oxidative signaling, influencing metabolism. These bioactive compounds such as AsA, phenols, anthocyanins, flavonoids and carotenoids belong to the plant's defense system, and many of them have health-promoting effects in the prevention of cancer and cardiovascular diseases (Boeing et al. 2012; Haminiuk et al. 2012; Barbagallo et al. 2013). It is very useful to increase these bioactive compounds by a controlled abiotic stress such as RDI.

Through our research, we have checked the aforementioned hypothesis. For example, one of the main ROS compounds is H_2O_2. It is highly related to

CAT action. When concentration of H_2O_2 increases, enzymes such as CAT are activated. In our case, the higher the stress, the more CAT activity we could detect (Falagán et al. 2015b). In this sense, we also consider CAT to be a good indicator for water stress. Regarding the cited behavior of vitamin C with the degradation of AsA into DHA, we wanted to observe how APX, the enzyme involved in the process, acted against water stress. In the investigation carried out on peaches subjected to RDI strategies, APX uses AsA as electron donor to detoxify H_2O_2 as ROS which was over-produced during controlled drought (Falagán et al. 2015b).

To investigate more deeply the previous concept of the relationship between abiotic stress and the bioactive compound increase, we focused on phenylalanine ammoniolyase (PAL), a key enzyme which catalyzed the shikimic acid pathway L-phenlyalanine to produce *trans*-cinnamic acid. This compound leads to most of the phenolic compounds. Indeed, *trans*-cinnamic acid can be transformed into an intermediate product such as sinapic acid, coumaric acid, etc. which, in turn, leads to chlorogenic acid, for example. In our study, its isomer, neochlorogenic acid, was also clearly detected. Both chlorogenic and neochlorogenic acids are characteristic of peaches (Infante et al. 2011). Another health-promoting compound detected was caffeic acid. This compound also leads to chlorogenic acid because this ester is formed with caffeic acid and L-quinic acid (3-O-caffeoyl-D-quinic acid).

All these changes, depend on the duration and intensity of RDI, provoking a more or less strong response of the plant to water stress.

3. Postharvest Management

3.1. Whole Product

Stone fruit are highly perishable commodities, which leads to higher postharvest losses when compared with apples, pears or oranges. According to Tonini and Caccioni (1990), these losses are provoked by their high metabolism, which increase senescence processes, high sensibility to fungal attacks and high water losses due to transpiration. Some of them, such as transpiration, result in weight loss, shriveling and withering. To prevent this kind of damage, some techniques such as quick pre-cooling (generally using cold air) or cold (chilling) storage can be used. The use of controlled atmosphere (CA), modified atmosphere packaging, or other postharvest treatments in combination with low temperature can delay fruit deterioration

(Luchsinger and Artés 2000; Falagán et al. 2012; Vendrell and Carrasquer 1994).

a. Cold Storage

Food storage has always been an important issue for humans. Fruits and vegetables are alive after harvest, and it is necessary to decrease their respiratory activity and metabolism in order to delay ripening and senescence. Cold storage is the most practical way to delay metabolism and hence prolong shelf-life. Low temperature decreases enzymatic and microbial activities, reduces respiratory rate and vapor pressure deficit between the product and the atmosphere, reducing transpiration. It is essential to know the postharvest temperature tolerance of each commodity. Concretely, the optimum range for peaches and nectarines varies between -1 and +2ºC during 2-4 weeks for most cvs. (Fernández-Trujillo and Artés, 1998).

b. Controlled Atmosphere

Some postharvest techniques can help the action of cold storage and even prevent CI. One of these techniques is CA, which consists of atmosphere modification in hermetic storage chambers, lowering O_2 concentration and increasing CO_2, compared with the normal air atmosphere (21 KPa O_2 and 0.03 KPa CO_2) (Kader 1986). CA should be supplementary to temperature and RH management. Optimun ranges of temperature and RH should be maintained for each commodity during postharvest handling.

The effect of the atmosphere on peach and nectarine quality depends on the cv., gas rate, storage temperature, maturity stage of the fruit and postharvest treatments applied. Thompson (1996) reported that low O_2 concentrations reduced respiration rate and with the reduction of the oxidation substrate, the subsequently delay in climacteric fruit maturation (Lurie 1992; Retamales et al. 1992; Crisosto et al. 1995; Zhou et al. 2000). Initial recommendations for CA storage of peaches and nectarines were similar to those for some apple cvs.: 3–5% CO_2+ 1–2% O_2 at 0ºC (Anderson et al. 1969; Kader 1986). The changes in the atmosphere that surround the fruit tissue have effects on cellular metabolism. Thompson (2003) observed that the increase of CO_2 implied a reduction in synthesis reaction of climateric fruits, delaying senescence. Besides, the inhibition of some enzymatic reactions have been found, as well as a decrease in the production of volatile compounds.

One of the reasons for this delay in senescence is the inhibition of ethylene (C_2H_4), a key natural plant hormone synthetized in different parts of the plant such as leaves, stems, roots, flowers, fruits, tubers or seeds. C_2H_4 acts at trace levels throughout the life of the plant by stimulating or regulating the ripening of fruit, the opening of flowers or the abscission of leaves. C_2H_4 production is regulated by several developmental and environmental factors. Generally, C_2H_4 production is induced during certain phases of the plant cycle, including germination, ripening of fruits, and abscission of leaves and senescence of flowers. Some other factors can also affect the C_2H_4 production such as mechanical wounding, environmental stresses, and certain chemicals including auxin and other regulators (Yang and Hoffman 1984).

Biosynthesis of ethylene begins with the aminoacid methionine changing into S-adenosyl-L-methionine (SAM) due to the enzyme S-adenosylmethioninesynthetase, later converted to 1-aminocyclopropane-1-carboxylic acid (ACC) by the enzyme ACC synthase (ACS). The C_2H_4 production rate is determined by ACS activity. The final step requires O_2 and includes the enzyme ACC-oxidase. In this sense, a reduction in O_2 in the atmosphere inhibits C_2H_4 production, delaying senescence (Mathooko et al. 2001).

It is important to mention that high CO_2 concentrations in the CA inhibit ACC synthase activity, and as a consequence, the C_2H_4 production.

These processes impact on physical parameters which are related to quality, such as weight and firmness losses, highly related to ripening. Thanks to them we can detect maturation and deterioration. As explained earlier, the CA storage moderates the C_2H_4 production and respiration rate, slowing down senescence and its derived symptoms from cell wall degradation that lead to softening (Salmerón and Artés 1991; Artés et al. 1996; Kader 2007; Gwanpua 2012). This delay in senescence is also observed in skin color. In our studies, nectarines stored under CA maintained green color while those air-stored became redder with time (Falagán et al. 2015a). In this comparative study, we observed that SSC was not affected by postharvest handling. This content followed the typical decrease due to the consumption of sugars as respiratory substrates during climacteric fruit ripening and senescence, in stone fruit.

The modification of surrounding atmosphere during long-distance transport is widely used. Its application is essential in order to improve fresh horticultural product exportation.

c. 1-Methylcyclopropene

As previously mentioned, C_2H_4 is harmful to fruits during storage due to induction of softening, ripening and deterioration of fruit tissues (Dong et al. 2001). The C_2H_4 can diffuse into and out of plant tissues from both endogenous and exogenous sources. On the other hand, endogenous C_2H_4

production is indispensable for ripening processes. The C_2H_4 can be applied exogenously. For example, in banana it is a common procedure to make it ripen more quickly. However, normally, the objective is to delay senescence and because of that, the general strategy is to avoid the exposure to C_2H_4, or at least minimize it (Watkins 2002). In the last few years, C_2H_4 inhibitors have emerged. One promising example is the inhibitor for C_2H_4 perception: 1-methylcyclopropene (1-MCP), which interacts with C_2H_4 receptors and in this way, prevents C_2H_4-dependent responses (Sisler and Blankenship 1996; Sisler and Serek 1997, 2003). Other compounds have been shown to block the C_2H_4 binding site, causing an inhibition of C_2H_4 effects as 2,5-norbornadiene and diazocyclopentadiene, but neither of these compounds is commercially acceptable due to toxicity and manufacturing concerns (Fan et al. 1999). The 1-MCP is thought to fill C_2H_4 receptors such that C_2H_4 cannot bind and elicit action. The affinity of 1-MCP for the receptor is approximately 10 times greater than that of C_2H_4 (Blankenship and Dole 2003).

Commercialization of 1-MCP was first used for ornamental crops and undertaken by Floralife Inc. (Walterboro, SC). The product was approved by the United States Environmental Protection Agency in 1999 for ornamentals. Commercial application of 1-MCP to edible crops was undertaken by AgroFresh, Inc., under the trade name SmartFresh®. Diffusion of 1-MCP out of plant material is rapid. After 8 h of application, no 1-MCP was detected in the core area of individual apples (Blankenship and Dole 2003). In the case of sealed polyethylene bags, no measurable 1-MCP was distinguished in 15 days after introducing 1 $\mu L\ L^{-1}$ of 1-MCP to bananas (Jiang et al. 1999).

Regarding safety, toxicity and environmental profiles of 1-MCP concerning humans, animals and the environment are extremely favorable (Environmental Protection Agency, 2002). In general, 1-MCP is used at low rates, has a non-toxic mode of action and is chemically similar to naturally occurring substances (Blankenship and Dole 2003).

In peaches and nectarines, the recommended range of 1-MCP application is 20 $nL\ L^{-1}$; 0.1 $\mu L\ L^{-1}$; 0.5 $mL\ L^{-1}$during 12 to 24 h at 20-24°C (Dong et al. 2001; Mathooko et al. 2001; Fan et al. 2002). These authors noticed how 1-MCP maintained firmness and acidity, delayed C_2H_4 production and reduced respiration rate and also C_2H_4 associated enzymes and cell wall degrading enzymes. On the other hand, some prejudicial issues were detected, internal browning increased and juice was reduced. It is important to add to these recommendations the maturity stage of the fruit as a consideration. Besides, the time from harvest to 1-MCP treatment should be taken into account because the more perishable the crop, the more quickly after harvest 1-MCP should be applied (Blankenship and Dole 2003).

Some studies have shown that blocking C_2H_4 action with 1-MCP appeared to prevent normal ripening of several peaches and nectarines after cold storage (Dong et al. 2001). Peaches treated with 1-MCP were firmer than untreated fruit after 5°C storage. However, they showed more severe flesh browning than control fruit (Fan et al. 2002). Despite this, research has pointed out that C_2H_4 is essential for proper ripening of peaches and nectarines after storage (Blankenship and Dole 2003).

In our studies we have observed how 1-MCP-treatment of nectarines helped to maintain their antioxidant capacity and phenolic content. We attributed this fact to the 1-MCP ability to preventing the generation of free radicals (Falagán et al. 2015a).

3.2. Fresh-Cut Product

a. Concept

In the last few years, a large growth of the FC fruit and vegetable industry has been observed (Rico et al. 2007). Sociocultural changes have increased the intake of food which is easy to prepare and consume. The main reason is the global drive for healthier diet, searching for products that can delay aging and several diseases. Healthy, additive-free and environmentally respectful products are increasingly demanded. Besides, the increase of purchasing power has resulted in a demand for FC fruits and vegetables (Pérez et al. 2002). In this sense, retail marketing has led to an increase in the demand for FC, healthy and convenient food produce as previously mentioned (Caleb et al. 2013). FC products require little preparation time for the consumer and supply the same functional characteristics as the original whole commodity (Ahvenainen 1996, Artés and Allende 2005). Nowadays, catering and collective food services represent the greatest share of the demand for FC products. Nevertheless, it has more recently spread to supermarkets, restaurants and food stores (Artés et al. 2007).

These products consist of minimally processed fresh fruit and vegetables ready for consumption and only subjected to light intervention methods such as: washing, cutting, grating, shredding, leaf removal, etc. and packing at chilling temperatures under polymeric films (Artés and Allende 2005) commonly with a selective permeability to gas diffusion. Shewfelt (1987) adds to these operations the possible application of low irradiation levels. Other authors such as Wiley (1997) defined FC products as those commodities which maintain their tissues alive as well as those which have suffered little modification, including cold storage and controlled and modified atmospheres.

Fruit and vegetables are related to the concept of high functional quality without synthetic additives (Rico et al. 2007; Gialamas et al. 2010). Indeed, a considerable part of the vitamins and minerals that should be included in the diet, come from the consumption of fruit and vegetables (Caleb et al. 2013). However, it is known that processing of FC products induces a faster physiological deterioration, changes in bioactive compounds and risk of microbiological growth (O'Bernie and Francis 2003; Rico et al. 2007). These issues result in a fast degradation of organoleptic properties such us color, texture and flavour (Kabir 1994; Varoquaux and Wiley 1994), and finally in a microbial contamination of the commodity (Artés and Allende 2005).

b. General Procedures

The general quality condition, which includes, not only physical parameters but also functional facts, is affected by various factors. The most important factor is temperature (Watada and Qi 1999). Indeed, with increased respiration rate, deterioration increases at a comparable rate; thus, low temperature is essential for maintaining good quality. In this sense, every operation should be carried out at the appropriate temperature. If too cold, FC products are also sensible to CI, although their shelf-life is commonly shorter than the time lag for CI symptoms development.

In the following diagram, adapted from Silveira et al. (2015a), basic procedures are shown.

Ready-to-eat fruits and vegetables have their surfaces exposed to environment conditions due to cutting process besides being a rich matrix for microorganism growth (Azarakhsh et al. 2014). To prevent the proliferation of possible microorganisms, the majority of FC produce manufacturers use chlorine-based washing procedures (Artés et al. 2009). Despite this, during shelf-life, microbial counts may appear. Microorganisms can get to the fresh produce from different sources including postharvest handling and processing (Tomás-Callejas et al. 2012). This is why, after harvest and selection and quality control, whole product must be sanitized before the following operations. Huxsoll and Bolin (1989) suggested 5 to 10 L per fruit kg as the initial rinse to eliminate pesticide residues and other possible contamination. A water temperature below 5ºC is also recommended (Ahvenainen 1996). Then, chlorinated water dip should be considered in order to effectively reduce the microbial loads on the fruit surface (Soliva-Fortuny and Martín-Belloso 2003).

Chlorine is provided for the disinfection of the fruit surface by adding sodium hypoclorite (NaOCl) to the wash water. However, chlorine safety use has been questioned and, because of this, alternative ways of sanitizing FC fruits are needed (Aguayo et al. 2006).

The feasibility of hydrogen peroxide treatments (Silveira et al. 2008; Artés et al. 2009), organic acids such as peroxyacetic or octanoic acid (Silveira et al. 2011b; Wang and Ryser 2014), the use of irradiation (Beuchat et al.2001), ozone (Artés and Allende 2005; Aguayo et al. 2006; Aguayo et al. 2014), electrolyzed water (Artés-Hernández et al. 2014) or UV light treatment (Escalona et al. 2010) are some of the current options.

Peeling and cutting operations imply damage and stress in fruit tissues, as previously mentioned. Wounding stresses result in metabolic activation. This activation provokes an increase in respiration rate, and sometimes in C_2H_4 production (Varoquaux and Wiley 1994). Besides, membrane degradation and the subsequent cellular disruption and decompartmentalization of enzymes and substrates normally occur (Portela and Cantwell 2006). These events provoke reduction in quality characteristics, such as texture, color (mainly browning), flavor and even functional value and microbial deteroration (Cantwell 1992; Artés and Allende 2005; Artés et al. 2007). The intensity of wound response is affected by several factors as cv., maturity stage, temperature, O_2 and CO_2 concentrations, water vapor pressure, various inhibitors, and severity of wounding (Artés and Allende 2005; Portela and Cantwell 2006). To minimize injured tissues, very sharp cutting tools must be used and every process should be held in chilled conditions.

After cutting, a second wash is convenient in order to rinse the product. Later, some quality treatments can be applied. The need for additive use to help sanitizer action has become apparent. However, consumers have become more critical of the use of synthetic additives to preserve food safety or enhance characteristics such as color and flavor (Rico et al. 2007). To meet this demand, some studies have explored the application of natural compounds for healthier and higher quality FC products (Soliva-Fortuny and Martín-Belloso 2003; Pasha et al. 2014). Regarding consumer awareness of the use of chemically synthesized additives in food, natural antimicrobial agents have been introduced as a novel way to improve microbiological stability of FC fruit (Oms-Oliu et al. 2010).

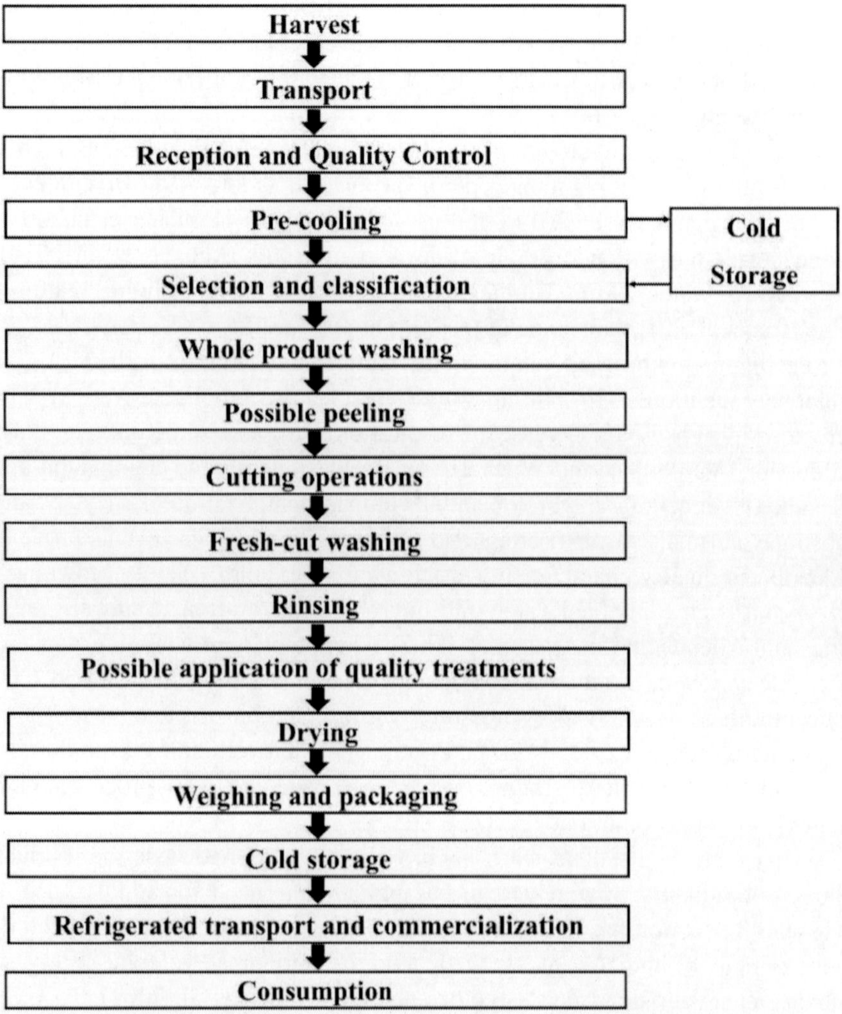

Figure 12. Flow diagram representing procedure steps for minimal processing.

Cinnamon and vanilla are popular and well-accepted flavors among consumers. They form part of many foods such as ice cream, beverages, biscuits, chocolate and other products (Raybaudi-Massilia et al. 2008). Their antimicrobial properties have been well known since antiquity, acting on different bacteria, yeasts and moulds (Bullerman 1974; Rojas-Graü et al. 2007; Muthuswamy et al. 2008; Raybaudi-Massilia et al. 2009; Silveira et al. 2015b).

Additives can also maintain visual and functional quality. For example, browning is also a major concern related to the extension of shelf-life of FC fruit and strongly affects consumer purchase decisions (Oms-Oliu et al. 2010). Reducing agents such as citric acid or ascorbic acid have been explored to prevent browning in FC products (Soliva-Fortuny et al. 2002; Aguayo et al. 2010). These kinds of additives also show antioxidant properties, as they are effective against the superoxide radical anion, hydrogen peroxide, hydroxyl radical, singlet oxygen and reactive nitrogen oxide (Barros et al. 2011). Besides, treatments that contain calcium maintain or improve tissue firmness and crispness. Calcium salts such as calcium lactate, calcium propionate or calcium ascorbate have been investigated as alternative sources of calcium (Alandes et al. 2006; Quiles et al. 2007; Aguayo et al. 2008; Silveira et al. 2011a). In this sense, surface treatments through applications such as dipping fruit pieces into aqueous solutions containing antimicrobial agents, antioxidants, calcium salts or functional ingredients such as minerals and vitamins have been widely studied to improve overall quality of FC fruit (Oms-Oliu et al. 2010). In this sense, Falagán et al. (2016) reported that the combination of an antibrowning agent such as calcium ascorbate and natural antimicrobials such as vanillin and cinnamic acid, helped to control microbiological growth of FC nectarines, maintaining quality parameters at a high level. This dipping is a 'green' alternative for organic FC products, compared to other chemical sanitizers such as chlorine.

4. Combining Postharvest Treatments and Deficit Irrigation Strategies

As previously mentioned, RDI induces a stress situation either for the tree or the final product, which implies an increase in some bioactive compound concentration and in SSC. However, the impact of this kind of irrigation strategy on postharvest behavior has not been deeply studied. In the case of nectarines and peaches, we have carried out several experiments in order to test if high postharvest quality is possible once the fruit have been subjected to RDI strategies.

So, regarding whole fruit: is it possible to maintain the higher quality achieved thanks to RDI stress? Do stone fruit ripen more quickly after being subjected to water deficit? From our experience, it is a promising combination. We observed that the better characteristics due to RDI were maintained during postharvest when stored under CA or treated with 1-MCP. As previously mentioned, some characteristics such as total phenols, antioxidant capacity and vitamin C slowed down their degradation produced by senescence when applying treatments such as CA and 1-MCP through the mechanisms previously explained. In this sense, found a more appealing product with proper firmness and flavor and more functionality even after the postharvest period, when compared with control samples.

Therefore, RDI can be used as a commercial field practice for extra early nectarines and peaches. It does not induce any limitation to postharvest handling while saving a great amount of water.

The same behavior was found when minimal processing was carried out. The main issues that a FC product faces are microbial counts and visual appearance problems related to dehydratation and browning, as previously mentioned. Neither of these processes was affected by RDI strategies, as we observed when compared with control sample behavior. The changes during storage were attributed to the consumption of organic acids as respiratory substrate for the fruit pieces (Falagán et al. 2015c). This progression is characteristic of climacteric fruits ripening and senescence (Kader 2002), such as in nectarines and peaches. In this sense, we consider RDI did not negatively affect the suitability of nectarines and peaches for FC processing.

References

Aguayo, E., Escalona, V. H. and Artés, F. (2006). Effect of cyclic exposure to ozone gas on physicochemical, sensorial and microbial quality of whole and sliced tomatoes. *Postharvest Biology and Technology*, *39*, 169-177.

Aguayo, E., Escalona, V. H. and Artés, F. (2008). Effect of hot water treatment and various calcium salts on quality of fresh-cut 'amarillo' melon. *Postharvest Biology and Technology*, *47*, 397-406.

Aguayo, E., Escalona, V. H., Silveira, A. C. and Artés, F. (2014). Quality of tomato slices disinfected with ozonated water. *Food Science and Technology International*, *20*, 227-235.

Aguayo, E., Requejo-Jackman, C., Stanley, R. and Woolf, A. (2010). Effects of calcium ascorbate treatments and storage atmosphere on antioxidant activity and quality of fresh-cut apple slices. *Postharvest Biology and Technology*, *57*, 52-60.

Ahvenainen, R. (1996). New approaches in improving the shelf life of minimally processed fruit and vegetables. *Trends in Food Science and Technology*, *7*, 179-187.

Alandes, L., Hernando, I., Amparo, Quiles., Pérez-Munuera, I. and Lluch, M. A. (2006). Cell wallstability of fresh-cut Fuji apples treated with calcium lactate. *Journal of Food Science*, *71*, 615-620.

Alvisi, F., Malagoli, C., Pirazzoli, C. and Regazzi, D. (1995). Economic aspect of peach growing in the mediterranean area. Medit. *(CIHEAM-IAMB)*, *6*, 35-38.

Anderson, R. E., Parsons, C. S. and Smith, W. L. (1969). Controlled atmosphere storage of Eastern-grown peaches and nectarines. Agricultural Research Service, U.S. Dept. of Agriculture, Washington, D.C.

Anon, L. (2008). Peach. In: Goldman, L., Hobson, A., Norton, S. R. (Eds), The Columbia Electronic Encyclopedia, 6th Edition. Columbia University Press, New York.

Anttonen, M. J. and Karjalainen, R. O. (2005). Environmental and genetic variation of phenolic compounds in red raspberry. *Journal of Food Composition and Analysis*, *18*, 759-769.

Artés, F. (2000). Productos vegetales procesados en fresco, in: Lamúa, M. (Ed.), Aplicación del Frío a los Alimentos. Mundi Prensa 5, Spain, 127-141.

Artés, F., Mínguez, M. I. and Hornero, D. (2002). Analysing changes in fruit pigments. In: Colour in Food. Improving Quality. Ed. D. B. Mac Dougall. Edit. CRC Press and Woodhead Publishing Ltd. Cambridge, UK. Chapter 10. 248-282.

Artés, F. and Allende, A. (2005). Minimal fresh processing of vegetables, fruits and juices, in: Sun, D. W. (Ed.), *Emerging technologies for food processing*, *26*, Spain, 677-716.

Artés, F., Cano, A. and Fernández-Trujillo, J. P. (1996). Pectolytic enzyme activities during intermittent warming storage of peaches. *Journalof the Food Science*, *61*, 2, 311-313.

Artés, F., Gómez, P. A. and Artés-Hernández, F. (2007). Physical, physiological and microbial deterioration of minimally fresh processed fruits and vegetables. *Food Science and Technology International*, *13*, 177-188.

Artés, F., Gómez, P., Aguayo, E., Escalona, V. and Artés-Hernández, F. (2009). Sustainable sanitation techniques for keeping quality and safety of fresh-cut plant commodities. *Postharvest Biology and Technology*, *51*, 287-296.

Artés-Hernández, F., Gómez, P., Aguayo, E., Tomás-Callejas, A. and Artés, F. (2014). Sustainable Processing of Fresh-Cut Fruit and Vegetables, in:

Tiwari B. K., Norton T., Holden, N. M. (Eds.), Sustainable Food Processing. *John Wiley and Sons*, Ltd, 219-268.

Azarakhsh, N., Osman, A., Ghazali, H. M., Tan, C. P. and Adzahan, N. M. (2014). Lemongrass essential oil incorporated into alginate-based edible coating for shelf-life extension and quality retention of fresh-cut pineapple. *Postharvest Biology and Technology*, *88*, 1-7.

Badenes, M. L., Llácer, G. and Crisosto, C. H. (2006). Mejora de la Calidad de Frutales de Hueso, in: Llácer, G., Díez, M. J., Carrillo J. M., Badenes, M. L. (Eds.), Mejora genética de la calidad en plantas. Sociedad Española de Ciencias Hortícolas y Sociedad Española de Genética, Spain, 551-578.

Barbagallo, R. N., Di Silvestro, I. and Patanè, C. (2013). Yield, physicochemical traits, antioxidant pattern, polyphenol oxidase activity and total visual quality of field-grown processing tomato cv. Brigade as affected by water stress in Mediterranean climate. *Journal of the Science of Food and Agriculture*, *93*, 1449-1457.

Barros, A. I., Nunes, F. M., Gonçalves, B., Bennett, R. N. and Silva, A. P. (2011). Effect of cooking on total vitamin C contents and antioxidant activity of sweet chestnuts (*Castanea sativa* Mill.). *Food Chemistry*, *128*, 165-172.

Bassi, D. and Monet, R. (2008). Botany and Taxonomy. The peach: botany, production and uses. CAB International, United Kingdom.

Behboudian, M. H. and Mills, T. M. (1997). Deficit irrigation in deciduous orchards. *Horticultural Reviews*, *21*, 105-131.

Behboudian, M. H., Marsal, J., Girona, J. and López, G. (2011). Quality and yield responses of deciduous fruits to reduced irrigation. *Horticultural Reviews*, *38*,149-189.

Ben Mechlia, N., Ghrab, M., Zitouna, R., Ben Mimoun, M. and Masmoudi, M. (2002). Cumulative effect over five years of deficit irrigation on peach yield and quality. *Acta Horticulturae, 592*, 301-307.

Benvenuti, S., Pellati, F., Melegari, M. and Bertelli, D. (2004). Polyphenols, anthocyanins, ascorbic acid, and radical scavenging activity of Rubus, Ribes, and Aronia. *Journal of the Food Science*, *69*, 164-169.

Beuchat, L. R., Farber, J. M., Garrett, E. H., Harris, L. J., Parish, M. E., Suslow, T. V., Busta, F. F. (2001). Standardization of a method to determine the efficacy of sanitizers in inactivating human pathogenic microorganisms on raw fruits and vegetables. *Journal of Food Protection*, *64*, 1079-1084.

Blankenship, S. M. and Dole, J. M. (2003). 1-Methylcyclopropene: a review. *Postharvest Biology and Technology, 28*, 1-25.

Bleiholder, H., Van den Boom, T., Langeluddeke, P., Stauss, R. 1989. Einheitlichecodierung derphänologischenstadienbeikultur-und schadp-flanzen. *GesundePflanzen*, *41*, 381-384.

Boeing, H., Bechthold, A., Bub, A., Ellinger, S., Haller, D., Kroke, A., Leschik-Bonnet, E., Müller, M. J., Oberritter, H., Schulze, M., Stehle, P. and Watzl, B. (2012). Critical review: Vegetables and fruit in the prevention of chronic diseases. *European Journal of Nutrition*, *51*, 637-663.

Boland, A. M., Jerie, P. H., Mitchell, P. D. and Goodwin, I. (2000). Long-term effects of restricted root volume and regulated deficit irrigation on peach I. Growth and mineral nutrition. *Journal of the American Society for Horticultural Science*, *125*, 135-142.

Bolin, H. R. and Huxsoll, C. C. (1989). Storage stability of minimally processed fruit. *Journal of Food Biochemistry*, *13*, 281-292.

Bruhn, C. M., Feldman, N., Garlitz, C., Hardwood, J., Ivan, E., Marshall, M., Riley, A., Thurber, D. and Williamson, E. (1991). Consumer perceptions of quality: apricots, cantaloupes, peaches, pears, strawberries, and tomatoes. *Journal of Food Quality*, *14*, 187-195.

Bullerman, L. (1974). Inhibition of aflatoxin production by cinnamon. *Journal of Food Science*, *39*, 1163-1165.

Byrne, D. H. (2003). Breeding peaches and nectarines for mild-winter climate areas: state of the art and future directions, in: Marra, F., Sottile, F. (Eds.), Proceedings of the 1st Mediterranean Peach Symposium. *Agrigento, Italy*, 102-109.

Caleb, O. J., Mahajan, P. V., Al-Said, F. A. J. and Opara, U. L. (2013). Modified atmosphere packaging technology of fresh and fresh-cut produce and the microbial consequences - a review. *Food and Bioprocess Technology*, *6*, 303-329.

Cantwell, M. (1992). Postharvest handling systems: Minimally processed fruits and vegetables, in: Kader A. A. (Ed.), Postharvest technology of horticultural crops. 2nd Edition. University of California, *Division of Agriculture and Natural Resources*, *3311*, United States of America, 277-281.

Carusso, T. and Sottile, F. (1999). La peschicoltura autunnale in Sicilia: aspetti ambientali, varietali e colturali. *Frutticoltura*, *2*, 39-46.

Castrejón, A. D. R., Eichholz, I., Rohn, S., Kroh, L. W. and Huyskens-Keil, S. (2008). Phenolic profile and antioxidant activity of highbush blueberry (*Vaccinium corymbosum* L.) during fruit maturation and ripening. *Food Chemistry*, *109*, 564-572.

Čermák, J., Kučera, J., Baurerle, W. L., Phillip, N. and Hinckley, M. (2007). Tree water storage and its diurnal dynamics related to sap flow and changes in stem volume in old-growth Douglas-fir trees. *Tree Physiology*, *27*, 181-198.

Chalmers, D. J., Mitchell, P. D. and Jerie, P. H. (1983), July. The physiology of growth control of peach and pear trees using reduced irrigation. *In International Workshop on Controlling Vigor in Fruit Trees*, *146*, 143-150.

Cheng, G. W. and Crisosto, C. H. (1994). Development of dark skin discoloration on peach and nectarine fruit in response to exogenous contaminations. *Journal of the American Society for Horticultural Science*, *119*, 529-533.

Conejero, W., Mellisho, C. D., Ortuño, M. F., Moriana, A., Moreno, F. and Torrecillas, A. (2011). Using trunk diameter sensors for regulated deficit irrigation scheduling in early maturing peach trees. *Environmental and Experimental Botany*, *71*, 409-415.

Conesa, M. R., Domingo, R. and Pérez-Pastor, A. (2014). A new approach to ascertain the sensitivity to water stress of different plant water indicators in extra-early nectarine trees. *Scientia Horticulturae*, *169*, 147-153.

Corell, M., Girón, I. F., Galindo, A., Torrecillas, A., Torres-Sánchez, R., Pérez-Pastor, A., Moreno, F. and Moriana, A. (2014). Using band dendrometers in irrigation scheduling: Influence of the location inside the tree and comparison with point dendrometer. *Agricultural Water Management*, *142*, 29-37.

Crisosto, C. H., Johnson, R. S., Luza, J. G. and Crisosto, G. M. (1994). Irrigation regimes affect fruit soluble solids concentration and rate of waterloss of 'O'Henry' peaches. *HortScience*, *29*, 1169-1171.

Crisosto, C. H., Mitchell, F. G. and Johnson, R. S. (1995). Factors in fresh market stone fruit quality. *Postharvest News Information*, *5*, 17-21.

Crisosto, C. H., Mitchell, F. G. and Ju, Z. (1999). Susceptibility to chilling injury of peach, nectarine, and plum cultivars grown in California. *HortScience*, *34*, 1116-1118.

Crisosto, C. H. (2002). How do we increase peach consumption? *Acta Horticulturae*, *592*, 601-605.

Crisosto, C. H. and Labavitch, J. M. (2002). Developing a quantitative method to evaluate peach (*Prunus persica*) flesh mealiness. *Postharvest Biology and Technology*, *25*, 151-158.

Crisosto, C. (2006). Peach quality and postharvest technology. *Acta Horticulturae*, *713*, 479-487.

Escalona, V. H., Aguayo E., Martínez-Hernández, G. B. and Artés, F. (2010). Effect of UV-C on pathogen and spoilage bacterial growth in vitro and in inoculated baby spinach leaves. *Postharvest Biology and Technology*, *56*, 221-223.

Dangl, J. F., Dietrich, R. A. and Thomas, H. (2000). Senescence and programmed cell death, in: Buchanan, B., Gruissem, W., Jones, R. (Eds.), Biochemistry and molecular biology of plants. American Society of Plant Physiologist Press Rockville, United States of America, 1057, 1059.

De la Rosa, J. M., Conesa, M. R., Domingo, R., Torres, R. and Pérez-Pastor, A. (2013). Feasibility of using trunk diameter fluctuation and stem water potential reference lines for irrigation scheduling of early nectarine trees. *Agricultural Water Management*, *126*, 133-141.

Deslauriers, A., Morin, H., Urbinati, C. and Carrer, M. (2003). Daily weather response of balsam fir (*Abies balsamea* (L.) Mill.) stem radius increment from dendrometer analysis in the boreal forests of Québec (Canada). *Trees*, *17*, 477-484.

Dichio, B., Xiloyannis, C., Nuzzo, V., Montanaro, G. and Palese, A. M. (2004). Postharvest regulated deficit irrigation of peach tree in a Mediterranean environment: Effects on vegetative growth and yield. *Acta Horticulturae*, *664*, 169-174.

Dichio, B., Xiloyannis, C., Sofo, A. and Montanaro, G. (2007). Effects of post-harvest regulated deficit irrigation on carbohydrate and nitrogen partitioning, yield quality and vegetative growth of peach trees. *Plant and Soil*, *290*, 127-137.

Doltra, J., Oncins, J. A., Bonanay, J. and Cohen, M. (2007). Evaluation of plant-based water status indicators in mature apple trees under field conditions. *Irrigation Science*, *25*, 351-359.

Dong, L., Zhou, H., Sonego, L., Lers, A. and Lurie, S. (2001). Ethylene involvement in the cold storage disorder of 'Flavortop' nectarine. *Postharvest Biology and Technology*, *23*, 105-115.

Doorenbos, J. and Kassam, A. H. (1979). Yield response to water. *FAO Irrigation and Drainage Papers*, *33*. FAO, Rome, Italy.

Ehala, S., Vaher, M. and Kaljurand, M. (2005). Characterization of phenolic profiles of Northern European berries by capillary electrophoresis and determination of their antioxidant activity. *Journal of Agricultural and Food Chemistry*, *53*, 6484-6490.

Environmental Protection Agency. (2002). Federal Register, July 26. 67, 48796-48800.

Faci, J. M., Medina, E. T., Martínez-Cob, A. and Alonso, J. M. (2014). Fruit yield and quality response of a late season peach orchard to different irrigation regimes in a semi-arid environment. *Agricultural Water Management*, *143*, 102-112.

Falagán, N., Aguayo, E., Gómez, P. A., Artés-Hernández, F., Corbalán, M. and Artés, F. (2012). Combining deficit irrigation strategies and controlled atmosphere to maintain bioactive compounds in nectarine. *Acta Horticulturae*, *1012*, 97- 102.

Falagán, N., Artés, F. and Aguayo, E. (2016). Natural additives to preserve quality and improve nutritional value of fresh-cut nectarine. Food Science and Technology International, DOI: 1082013215621816.

Falagán, N., Artés, F., Gómez, P. A., Artés-Hernández, F., Conejero, W. and Aguayo, E. (2014). Deficit irrigation strategies combined with controlled atmosphere preserve quality in early peaches. *Food Science and Technology International*, *21*, 547-556.

Falagán, N., Artés, F., Artés-Hernández, F., Gómez, P. A., Pérez-Pastor, A. and Aguayo, E. (2015a). Comparative study on postharvest performance of nectarines grown under regulated deficit irrigation. *Postharvest Biology and Technology*, *110*, 24-32.

Falagán, N., Artés, F., Gómez, P. A., Artés-Hernández, F., Conejero, W. and Aguayo, E. (2015b). Deficit irrigation strategies enhance health-promoting compounds through the intensification of specific enzymes in early peaches. *Journal of the Science of Food and Agriculture*, DOI: 10.1002/jsfa.7290.

Falagán, N., Artés, F., Gómez, P. A., Artés-Hernández, F., Pérez-Pastor, A., de la Rosa, J. M. and Aguayo, E. (2015c). Combined effects of deficit irrigation and fresh-cut processing on quality and bioactive compounds of nectarines. *Horticultural Science*, *42*, 125-131.

Fan, X., Argenta, L. and Mattheis, J. P. (2002). Interactive effects of1-MCP and temperatures on 'Elberta' peach quality. *HortScience*, *37*, 134-138.

FAOSTAT. (2015). Statistical Databases. Food and Agriculture Organization of the United Nations. http://faostat3.fao.org/browse/Q/QC/E. (Accessed May, 2015).

Faust, M. (1989). Physiology of temperate zone fruit trees. John Wiley and Sons, Inc.

Fereres, E. and Soriano, M. A. (2007). Deficit irrigation for reducing agricultural water use. *Journal of Experimental Botany*, *58*, 147-159.

Fernández, J. E. and Cuevas, M. V. (2010). Irrigation scheduling from stem diameter variations: A review. *Agricultural and Forest Meteorology, 150*, 135-151.

Fernández-Trujillo, J. P. and Artés, F. (1997). Keeping quality of cold stored peaches using intermittent warming. *Food Research International, 30*, 441-450.

Fernández-Trujillo, J. P., Cano, A. and Artés, F. (1998). Physiological changes in peaches related to chilling injury and ripening. *Postharvest Biology and Technology, 13*, 109-119.

Geerts, A. and Raes, D. (2009). Deficit irrigation as an on-farm strategy to maximize crop water productivity in dry areas. *Agricultural Water Management, 96*, 1275-1284.

Geissler, C. (2009). The New Oxford Book of Food Plants. Oxford University Press, United Kingdom.

Gelly, M., Recasens, I., Girona, J., Mata, M., Arbones, A., Rufat, J. and Marsal, J. (2004). Effects of stage II and postharvest deficit irrigation on peach quality during maturation and after cold storage. *Journal of the Science of Food and Agriculture*, (*84*), 561-568.

Génard, M., Bertin, N., Borel, C., Bussières, P., Gautier, H., Habib, R., Léchaudel, M., Lecomte, A., Lescourret, F., Lobit, P. and Quilot, B. (2007). Towards a virtual fruit focusing on quality: modelling features and potential uses. *Journal of Experimental Botany*, (*58*), 917-928.

George, A. P. and Nissen, R. J. (1992). Effects of water stress, nitrogen and paclobutrazol on flowering, yield and fruit quality of the low-chill peach cultivar 'Flordaprince.' *Scientia Horticulturae, 49*, 197-209.

Ghrab, M., Sahli, A. and BenMechli, N. (1998). Reduction in vegetative growth and fruit quality improvement in the peach variety 'Carnival' through moderate watering restrictions. *Acta Horticulturae, 465*, 601-608.

Gialamas, H., Zinoviadou, K. G., Biliaderis, C. G. and Koutsoumanis, K. P. (2010). Development of a novel bioactive packaging based on the incorporation of *Lactobacillus sakei* into sodium-caseinate films for controlling *Listeria monocytogenes* in foods. *Food Research International, 43*, 2402-2408.

Goldhamer, D. A. (1989). Drought irrigation strategies for deciduous orchards. Cooperative extension. University of California, *Division of agricultural and natural resources, 21453*, pp. 15.

Goldhamer, D. A., Fereres, E., Mata, M., Girona, J. and Cohen, M. (1999). Sensitivity of continuous and discrete plant and soil water status monitoring in peach tress subjected to deficit irrigation. *Journal of the American Society for Horticultural Science*, *124*, 437-444.

Goldhamer, D. A. and Fereres, E. (2001). Irrigation scheduling protocols using continuously recorded trunk diameter measurements. *Irrigation Science*, *20*,115-125.

Goldhamer, D. A. and Fereres, E. (2004). Irrigation scheduling of almond trees with trunk diameter sensors. *Irrigation Science*, *23*, 11-19.

Goldhamer, D. A., Viveros, M. and Salinas, M. (2006). Regulated deficit irrigation in almonds: effects of variations in applied water and stress timing on yield and yield components. *Irrigation Science*, *24*, 101-114.

Gwanpua, S. G., Verlinden, B. E., Hertog, M. L. A. T. M., Bulens, I., Van de Poel, B., Van Impe, J., Nicolaï, B. M. and Geeraerd, A. H. (2012). Kinetic modeling of firmness breakdown in 'Braeburn'apples stored under different controlled atmosphere conditions. *Postharvest Biology and Technology*, *67*, 68-74.

Haffner, K., Rosenfeld, H. J., Skrede, G. and Wang, L. (2002). Quality of red raspberry *Rubus idaeus* L. cultivars after storage in controlled and normal atmospheres. *Postharvest Biology and Technology*, *24*, 279-289.

Haminiuk, C. W. I., Maciel, G. M., Plata-Oviedo, M. S. V. and Peralta, R. M. (2012). Phenolic compounds in fruits - an overview. *International Journal of Food Science and Technology*, *47*, 2023-2044.

Harborne, J. B. and Williams, C. A. (2000). Advances in flavonoid research since 1992. *Phytochemistry*, *55*, 481-504.

Harding, P. L. and Haller, M. H. (1934). Peach storage with special reference to breakdown. *Proceedings of the American Society for Horticultural Science*, *32*, 160-163.

Heim, K. E., Tagliaferro, A. R. and Bobilya, D. J. (2002). Flavonoid antioxidants: chemistry, metabolism and structure-activity relationships. *The Journal of Nutritional Biochemistry*, *13*, 572-584.

Hilaire, C. and Mathieu, V. (2004). Test hédoniques Sur variétés de pèche. D'abord, satisfaire le consommateur. *Infos-Centre Technique Interprofessionnel des Fruits et Légumes*, 32-35.

Hinckley, T. M. and Bruckerhoff, D. N. (1975). The effect of drought on water relations and stem shrinkage of *Quercus alba*. *Canadian Journal of Botany*, *53*, 62-72.

Hölttä, T., Linkosalo, T., Riikonen, A., Sevanto, S. and Nikinmaa, E. (2015). An analysis of Granier sap flow method, its sensitivity to heat storage and a new approach to improve its time dynamics. *Agricultural and Forest Meteorology*, *211*, 2-12.

Huguet, J. G., Li, S. H., Lorendeau, J. Y. and Pelloux, G. (1992). Specific micromorphometric reactions of fruit trees to water stress and irrigation scheduling automation. *Journal of Horticultural Science*, *67*, 631-640.

Iglesias, I., Carbó, J., Bonany, J., Casals, M., Dalmau, R. and Montserrat, R. (2005). Innovaciónvarietal en melocotonero: especial referencia a las nuevas variedades de nectarina. Fruticultura Profesional: *Especial Melocotonero III*, *152*, 6-36.

Iglesias, I., Carbó, J., Bonany, J. and Montserrat, R. (2007). Nuevas variedades de nectarina decarne blanca. *Vida Rural: Especial melocotonero II*, *244*, 19-21.

Iglesias, I. and Echeverría, G. (2009). Differential effect of cultivar and harvest date onnectarine color, quality and consumer acceptance. *Scientia Horticulturae*, *120*, 41-50.

Iglesias, I. (2010a). La coltivazione del pesco in Spagna: situazione produttiva, innovazioni varietali e tecniche colturali. *Italus Hortus*, *17*, 7-10.

Iglesias, I., Reig, G., Montserrat, R., Carbó, J. and Bonany, J. (2010b). Innovación varietal ennectarina y melocotón plano o paraguayo. Revista de Fruticultura: *Especialmelocotonero, nectarina y paraguayo*, *9*, 4-17.

Iglesias, I. (2013). Peach production in Spain: current situation and trends, from production to consumption, in: *Proceedings of the 4th Conference, Innovations in Fruit Growing*, 75-96.

Infante, R., Contador, L., Rubio, P., Aros, D. and Peña-Neira, Á. (2011). Postharvest sensory and phenolic characterization of 'Elegant Lady' and 'Carson'peaches. *Chilean Journal of Agricultural Research*, (*71*), 445-451.

Intrigliolo, D. S. and Castel, J. R. (2004). Continuous measurement of plant and soil water status for irrigation scheduling in plum. *Irrigation Science*, *23*, 93-102.

Intrigliolo, D. S. and Castel, J. R. (2007). Crop load affects maximum daily trunkshrinkage of plum trees. *Tree Physiology*, *27*, 89-96.

Jiang, Y., Joyce, D. C. and Macnish, A. J. (1999). Extension of the shelf life of banana fruit by 1-methylcyclopropene in combination with polyethylene bags. *Postharvest Biology and Technology*, *6*, 187-193.

Jiménez, S., Pinochet, J., Romero, J., Gogorcena, Y., Moreno, M. A. and Espada, J. L. (2011). Performance of peach and plum based rootstocks of different vigour on a late peach cultivar in replant and calcareous conditions. *Scientia Horticulturae*, *129*, 58-63.

Johnson, R. S., Handley, D. F. and DeJong, T. M. (1992). Long-term response of early maturing peach trees to postharvest water deficits. *Journal of the American Society for Horticultural Science*, *117*, 881-886.

Kabir, H. (1994). Fresh-cut vegetables, in: Brods, A. L., Herndon, V. A. (Eds.), Modified atmosphere food packaging. Institute of Packaging Professionals, United States of America, 155-160.

Kader, A. A. (1986). Biochemical and physiological basis for effects of controlled and modified atmospheres on fruits and vegetables. *Food Technology*, *40*, 99-104.

Kader, A. A. (2002). Postharvest Technology of Horticultural Crops, 3rd Ed. University of California, ANR Publication, 3311.

Kader, A. A. (Ed.). (2007). Tecnología postcosecha de cultivos hortofrutícolas. UCANR Publications.

Katerji, N., Mastrorilli, M. and Rana, G. (2008). Water use efficiency of cropscultivated in the Mediterranean region: Review and analysis. *European Journal of Agronomy*, *28*, 493-507.

Knox, J. W., Kay, M. G. and Weatherhead, E. K. (2012). Water regulation, crop production, and agricultural water management - Understanding farmer perspectives on irrigation efficiency. *Agricultural Water Management*, *108*, 3-8.

Kramer, A. and Twigg, V. B. A. (1966). Fundamentals of quality control for the food industry, 2nd Edition. Aci Publishing, Ireland.

Laribi, A. I., Palou, L., Intrigliolo, D. S., Nortes, P. A., Rojas-Argudo, C., Taberner, V., Bartual, J. and Pérez-Gago, M. B. (2013). Effect of sustained and regulated deficit irrigation on fruit quality of pomegranate cv. 'Mollar de Elche' at harvest and during cold storage. *Agricultural Water Management*, *125*, 61-70.

Larson, K. D., DeJong, T. M. and Johnson, R. S. (1988). Physiological and growth responses of mature peach trees to postharvest water stress. *Journal of the American Society for Horticultural Science*, *113*, 296-300.

Layne, R. E. C. and Tan, C. S. (1984). Long-term influence of irrigation and tree density on growth, survival, and production of peach. *Journal of the American Society for Horticultural Science*, *109*, 795-799.

Li, S. H., Huguet, J. G. and Bussi, C. (1989). Irrigation scheduling in mature tree peach orchard using tensiometers and dendrometers. *Irrigation and Drainage Systems*, *3*, 1-12.

Li, S. H., Huguet, J. G., Schoch, P. G. and Orlando, P. (1989). Response of peach-tree growth and cropping to soil water deficit at various phenological stages of fruit development. *Journal of Horticultural Science*, *64*, 541-552.

López, G., Girona, J. and Marsal, J. (2007). Response of winter root starch concentration to severe water stress and fruit load and its subsequent effects on early peach fruit development. *Tree Physiology*, *27*, 1619-1626.

Luchsinger, L. and Artés, F. (2000). Alleviating chilling injuries in stone fruit. In: Improving Postharvest Technologies for Fruits, Vegetables and Ornamentals. International Conference International Institute of Refrigeration. Murcia.

Lurie, S. (1992). Modified atmosphere storage of peaches and nectarines to reduce storage disorders. *International Journal of Food Science and Technology*, *27*, 507-514.

Lurie, S. and Crisosto, C. H. (2005). Chilling injury in peach and nectarine. *Postharvest Biology and Technology*, *37*, 195-208.

MAGRAMA. (2015). Statistical Databases. Ministerio de Agricultura, Alimentación y Medio Ambiente. http://www.magrama.gob.es. (Accessed May, 2015).

Marsham, R. (1759). Observations on the growth of trees. *Philosophical Transactions of the Royal Society*, *51*, 7-12.

Martínez-Calvo, J., Llácer, G., Cunill, M., Duran, S. and Badenes, M. L. (2006). Programa de mejora de melocotonero del IVIA. *Acta Horticulturae*, *45*, 221-222.

Mathooko, F. M., Tsunashima, Y., Owino, W. Z. O., Kubo, Y. and Inaba, A. (2001). Regulation of genes encoding ethylene biosynthetic enzymes in peach (*Prunus persica* L.) fruit by carbon dioxide and 1-methylcyclopropene. *Postharvest Biology and Technology*, *21*, 265-281.

Mercier, V., Bussi, C., Lescourret, F. and Génard, M. (2009). Effects of different irrigation regimes applied during the final stage of rapid growth on an early maturing peach cultivar. *Irrigation Science*, *27*, 297-306.

Mills, T. M., Behboudian, M. H., Tan, P. Y. and Clothier, B. E. (1994). Plant water status and fruit quality in 'Braeburn' apples. *HortScience 29*, 1274-1278.

Mitchell, F. G., Mayer, G., Biasi, W., Gulli, D. and Faubian, D. (1990). Selecting and handling high quality stone fruit, in: 1989 research reports for California peaches and nectarines. United States of America, pp. 15.

Mitchell, P. D. and Chalmers, D. J. (1982). The effect of reduced water supply on peach tree growth and yields. *Journal of the American Society for Horticultural Science*, *107*, 853-856.

Mitchell, P. D., Jerie, P. H. and Chalmers, D. J. (1984). The effects ofregulated water deficits on pear tree growth, flowering, fruit growth, and yield. *Journal of the American Society for Horticultural Science*, *109*, 604-606.

Mitchell, P. D., Chalmers, D. J., Jerie, P. H. and Burge, G. (1986). The use of initial withholding of irrigation and tree spacing to enhance the effect of regulated deficit irrigation on pear trees. *Journal of the American Society for Horticultural Science*, *111*, 858-861.

Mitchell, P. D., van den Ende, B., Jerie, P. H. and Chalmers, D. J. (1989). Responses of 'Barlett' pear to withholding irrigation, regulateddeficit irrigation, and tree spacing. *Journal of the American Society for Horticultural Science*, *114*, 15-19.

Moreno, M. A. (2005). Selección de patrones y variedades de meloctonero. Dossier frutales de hueso. Vida Rural Abril, 28-31.

Moriana, A., Fereres, E., Orgaz, F., Castro, Humanes, M. D. and Pastor, M. (2000). The relations between trunk diameter fluctuations and tree water status in olive trees (*Olea europea* L). *Acta Horticulturae*, *537*, 293-297.

Moriana, A. and Fereres, E. (2002). Plant Indicators for scheduling irrigation for young olive trees. *Irrigation Science*, *21*, 83-90.

Mounzer, O. H., Conejero, W., Nicolás, E., Abrisqueta, I., García-Orellana, Y. V., Tapia, L. M., Vera, J., Abrisqueta, J. M. and Ruiz-Sánchez, M. C. (2008). Growth pattern and phenological stages of early-maturing peach trees under a Mediterranean climate. *HortScience*, *43*, 1813-1818.

Mpelasoka, B. S., Behboudian, M. H. and Mills, T. M. (2001). Effects of deficit irrigation on fruit maturity and quality of 'Braeburn' apple. *Scientia Horticulturae*, *90*, 279-290.

Muthuswamy, S. and Rupasinghe, H. P. V. (2007). Fruit phenolics as antimicrobial agents: selective antimicrobial effect of catechin, chlorogenic acid, and phloridzin. *Journal of Food Agriculture and Environment*, *5*, 81-85.

Naor, A. (2001). Irrigation and crop load influence fruit size and water relations in field-grown 'Spadona' pear. *Journal of the American Society for Horticultural Science*, *126*, 252-255.

Naor, A. and Cohen, S. (2003). Sensitivity and variability of maximum trunk shrinkage, midday stem water potential, and transpiration rate inresponse to withholding irrigation from field grown apple trees. *HortScience*, *38*, 547-551.

Naor, A. (2006). Irrigation scheduling and evaluation of tree water status in deciduous orchards. *Horticultural Reviews*, *32*, 111-116.

Nunes, M. C. N. and Emond, J. P. (2002). Quality curves for two different peach cultivarsas a function of the storage temperature. Scientific report presented to Envirotainer, Sweden by the Air Cargo Transportation Research Group, University Laval, Quebec, Canada.

O'Beirne, D. and Francis, G. A. (2003). Reducing the pathogen risk in MAP-prepared produce, in: Ahvenainen, R. (Ed.), Novel food packaging techniques. Woodhead Publishing Limited/CRC Press LLC, United Kingdom, 231-286.

Oliveira, C. M. and Priestley, C. A. (1988). Carbohydrate reserves in deciduous fruit trees. *Horticultural Reviews*, *10*, 403-430.

Oms-Oliu, G., Rojas-Graü, M. A., González, L. A., Varela, P., Soliva-Fortuny, R., Hernando, M. I. H., Pérez, I., Fiszman, S. and Martín-Belloso, O. (2010). Recent approaches using chemical treatments to preserve quality of fresh-cut fruit: A review. *Postharvest Biology and Technology*, *57*, 139-148.

Ortuño, M. F., García-Orellana, Y., Conejero, W., Ruiz-Sánchez, M. C., Mounzer, O., Alarcón, J. J. and Torrecillas, A. (2006). Relationships between climatic variables and sap flow, stem water potential and maximum daily trunk shrinkage in lemon trees. *Plant and Soil*, *279*, 229-242.

Ortuño, M. F., Conejero, W., Moreno, F., Moriana, A., Intrigliolo, D. S., Biel, C., Mellisho, C. D., Pérez-Pastor, A., Domingo, R., Ruiz-Sánchez, M. C., Casadesus, J., Bonany, J. and Torrecillas, A. (2010). Could trunkdiameter sensors be used in woody crops for irrigation scheduling? A review of current knowledge and future perspectives. *Agricultural Water Management*, *97*, 1-11.

Parker, D., Ziberman, D., Moulton, K. (1991). How quality relates to price in California fresh peaches. *California Agriculture*, *45*, 14-16.

Pasha, I., Saeed, F., Sultan, M. T., Khan, M. R. and Rohi, M. (2014). Recent developments in minimal processing: a tool to retain nutritional quality of food. *Critical Reviews in Food Science and Nutrition*, *54*, 340-351.

Pereira, L. S., Cordery, I. and Iacovides, I. (2002). Coping with water scarcity. *Technical Documents in Hydrology*, *58*. UNESCO, Paris.

Pereira, L. S., Cordery, I. and Iacovides, I. (2012). Improved indicators of water use performance and productivity for sustainable water conservation and saving. *Agricultural Water Management*, *108*, 39-51.

Pérez, S., Cháfer, M. and Ortolá, M. D. (2002). Elaboración y factores de calidad en ensaladas procesadas en fresco. *Alimentaria*, *11*, 77-85.

Pérez-Pastor, A., Ruiz-Sánchez, M. C., Martínez, J. A., Nortes, P. A., Artés, F. and Domingo, R. (2007). Effect of deficit irrigation on apricot fruit quality at harvest and during storage. *Journal of the Science of Food and Agriculture*, *87*, 2409-2415.

Poiroux-Gonord, F., Bidel, L. P. R., Fanciullino, A. L., Gautier, H., López-Lauri, F. and Urban, L. (2010). Health benefits of vitamins and secondary metabolites of fruits and vegetables and prospects to increase their concentrations by agronomic approaches. *Journal of Agricultural and Food Chemistry*, *58*, 12065-12082.

Portela, S. I. and Cantwell, M. I. (2001). Cutting blade sharpness affects appearance and other quality attributes of fresh-cut cantaloupe melon. *Journal of Food Science*, *66*, 1265-1270.

Puig, C. P, Dagar, A., Marti Ibañez, C., Singh, V., Crisosto, C. H., Friedman, H., Lurie, S. and Granell, A. (2015). Pre-symptomatic transcriptome changes during cold storage of chilling sensitive and resistant peach cultivars to elucidate chilling injury mechanisms. *BMC Genomics*, *16*, 245-275.

Quiles, A., Hernando, I., Pérez-Munuera, I. and Lluch, M. A. (2007). Effect of calciumpropionate on the microstructure and pectin methylesterase activity in theparenchyma of fresh-cut Fuji apples. *Journal of the Science of Food and Agriculture*, *87*, 511-519.

Raybaudi-Massilia, R. M., Mosqueda-Melgar, J., Soliva-Fortuny, R. and Martin-Belloso, O. (2009). Control of pathogenic and spoilage microorganisms in fresh-cut fruitsand fruit juices by traditional and alternative natural antimicrobials. *Comprehensive Reviews in Food Science and Food Safety*, *8*, 157-180.

Retamales, J., Cooper, T., Streif, J. and Kama, J. C. (1992). Preventing cold storage disorders in nectarines. *Journal of Horticultural Science*, *67*, 619-626.

Rice-Evans, C. A., Miller, N. J., Bolwell, P. G., Bramley, P. M. and Pridham, J. B. (1995). The relative antioxidant activities of plant-derived polyphenolic flavonoids. *Free Radical Research*, *22*, 375-383.

Rico, D., Martín-Diana, A. B., Barat, J. M. and Barry-Ryan, C. (2007). Extending and measuring the quality of fresh-cut fruit and vegetables: a review. *Trends in Food Science and Technology*, *18*, 373-386.

Rojas-Graü, M. A., Raybaudi-Massilia, R. M., Soliva- Fortuny, R. C., Avena-Bustillos, R. J., McHugh, T. H. and Martín-Belloso, O. (2007). Apple puree-alginate edible coating as carrier of antimicrobial agents to prolong shelf-life offresh-cut apples. *Postharvest Biology and Technology*, *45*, 254-264.

Ruiz-Sánchez, M. C., Egea, J., Galego, R. and Torrecillas, A. (1999). Floral biology of Búlida apricot trees subjected to postharvest water irrigation withholding. *Annals of Applied Biology's*, *135*, 523-528.

Salmerón, M. C. and Artés, F. (1991). Parámetros físico-químicos y actividades enzimáticas pectinmetilesterasa y poligalacturonasa para melocotón Maruja y nectarina Armking bajo tratamientos de atmósfera controlada. *Agrochimica XXXV*, *4*, 289-297.

Schiermeier, Q. (2014). Water risk as world warms. *Nature*, *505*, 10.

Sevanto, S., Vesala, T., Perämäki, M. and Nikinmaa, E. (2002). Time lags for xylem and stem diameter variations in a Scots pine tree. *Plant Cell and Environment*, *25*, 1071-1077.

Shackel, K. (2000). The relation of midday stem water potential to the growth and physiology of fruit trees under water limited conditions. *Acta Horticulturae*, *537*, 425-430.

Shackel, K. A., Ahmadi, H., Biasi, W., Buchner, R., Goldhamer, D., Gurusinghe, S., Hasey, J., Kester, D., Krueger, B., Lampinen, B., McGourty, G., Micke, W., Mitcham, E., Olson, B., Pelletrau, K., Philips, H., Ramos, D., Schwankl, L., Sibbett, S., Snyder, R.,Soutwick, S., Stevenson, M., Thorpe, M., Weinbaum, S. and Yeager, J. (1997). Plant water status as an index of irrigation need in deciduous fruit trees. *HortTechnology*, *7*, 23-29.

Shewfelt, R. L. (1987). Quality of minimally processed fruits and vegetables. *Journal of Food Quality*, *10*, 143-156.

Siddiq, M., Liavoga, A. and Greiby, I. (2012). Peaches and Nectarines, in Sinha, N., Sidhu, J., Barta, J., Wu, J., Cano, M. P. (Eds.), Handbook of Fruits and Fruit Processing, 2nd Edition, 535-549.

Silveira, A. C., Aguayo, E., Chisari, M. and Artés, F. (2011a). Calcium salts and heat treatment for quality retention of fresh-cut 'Galia' melon. *Postharvest Biology and Technology*, *62*, 77-84.

Silveira, A. C., Aguayo, E., Escalona, V. H. and Artés, F. (2011b). Hot water treatment and peracetic acid to maintain fresh-cut 'Galia' melon quality. *Innovative Food Science and Emerging Technologies*, *12*, 569-576.

Silveira, A. C., Bustamante-Pezoa, A., Escalona, V. H. and Aguayo, E. (2015a). Quality preservation and safety of minimally processed vegetables, in: Hui, Y. H., ÖzgülEvranuz, E. (Eds.), Handbook of Vegetable Preservation and Processing. 2nd CRC Press, Taylor and Francis, Inc., Boca Raton, Florida, United States of America, 319-348.

Silveira, A. C., Conesa, A., Aguayo, E. and Artés, F. (2008). Alternative sanitizers to chlorine for use on fresh-cut 'Galia' (*Cucumis melo* var. *catalupensis*) melon. *Journal of Food Science*, *73*, 405-411.

Silveira, A. C., Moreira, G., Artés, F. and Aguayo, E. (2015b). Vanillin and cinnamic acid in aqueous solutions or in active modified packaging preserve the quality of fresh-cut Cantaloupe melon. *Scientia Horticulturae*, *192*, 271-278.

Singh, A., Patel, R. K., Babu, K. D. and De, L. C. (2007). 'Low chiling peaches.' Under utilized and under exploited horticultural crops. New Delhi: New India Publishing. pp. 90, India.

Sisler, E. C. and Blankenship, S. M. (1996). Methods of counter acting an ethylene response in plants, U.S.

Sisler, E. C. and Serek, M. (1997). Inhibitors of ethylene responses in plants at the receptor level: recent developments. *Physiologia Plantarum*, *100*, 577-582.

Sisler, E. C. and Serek, M. (2003). Compounds interacting with the ethylene receptor in plants. *Plant Biology*, *5*, 473-480.

Soliva-Fortuny, R. C., Oms-Oliu, G. and Martín-Belloso, O. (2002). Effects of ripeness stages on the storage atmosphere, color, and textural properties of minimally processed apple slices. *Journal of Food Science*, *67*, 1958-1963.

Soliva-Fortuny, R. C. and Martín-Belloso, O. (2003). New advances in extending the shelf-life of fresh-cut fruits: a review. *Trends in Food Science and Technology*, *14*, 341-353.

Spínola, V., Llorent-Martínez, E. J. and Castilho, P. C. (2014). Determination of vitamin C in foods: Current state of method validation. *Journal of Chromatography A*, *1369*, 2-17.

Stewart, J. I., Cuenca, R. H., Pruitt, W. O., Hagan, R. M. and Tosso, J. (1977). Determination and Utilization of water production functions for principal California crops. W-67 Calif. Contrib. Proj. Rep. University of California, Davis.

Szajdek, A. and Borowska, E. J. (2008). Bioactive compounds and health-promoting properties of berry fruits: a review. *Plant Foods for Human Nutrition*, *63*, 147-156.

Taylor, H. M., Jordan, W. R. and Sinclair, T. R. (1983). Limitations to efficient water use in crop production. American Society of Agronomy, Crop Society of America, Soil Science Society of America, United States of America.

Thacker, C. (1985). The history of gardens. Berkeley: University of California Press, United States of America.

Thompson, A. K. (1996). Postharvest Technology of fruit and Vegetables. Blackwell Publishing, United Kingdom.

Tiang, L., Canli, F. A., Wang, X. and Sibbald, S. (2009). Genetic transformation of *Prunus domestica* L. using the *hpt* gene coding for hygromycin resistance as the selectable marker. *Scientia Horticulturae*, *119*, 339-343.

Tomás-Callejas, A., López-Gálvez, F., Sbodio, A., Artés, F., Artés-Hernández, F. and Suslow, T. V. (2012). Chlorine dioxide and chlorine effectiveness to prevent *Escherichia coli* O157: H7 and *Salmonella* cross-contamination on fresh-cut Red Chard. *Food Control*, *23*, 325-332.

Torrecillas, A., Domingo, R., Galego, R. and Ruiz-Sánchez, M. C. (2000). Apricot tree response to withholding irrigation at different phenological periods. *Scientia Horticulturae*, *85*, 201-215.

Turner, N. C. (1981). Techniques and experimental approaches for the measurement of plant water status. *Plant and Soil*, *58*, 339-366.

Ueda, M. and Shibata, E. (2001). Diurnal changes in branch diameter as indicator of water status of Hinoki cypress, *Chamaecyparis obtuse. Trees*, *15*, 315-318.

Urban, L., Staudt, M., Ripoll, J., Lauri-López, F. and Bertin, N. (2014). Less can make more - Revisiting fleshy fruit quality and irrigation in horticulture. *Chronica Horticulturae*, *54*, 25-30.

Vallverdú, X., Girona, J., Echeverria, G., Marsal, J., Behboudian, M. H. and López, G. (2012). Sensory quality and consumer acceptance of 'Tardibelle'peach are improved by deficit irrigation applied during stage II of fruit development. *HortScience*, *47*, 656-659.

Varoquaux, P. and Wiley, R. (1994). Biological and biochemical changes in minimally processed refrigerated fruits and vegetables, in: Wiley, R. C. (Ed.), Minimally processed refrigerated fruits and vegetables. *Chapman and Hall*, United States of America, 226-268.

Vendrell, M. and Carrasquer, A. M. (1994). Fisiología poscosecha en frutos de hueso, in Vendrell, M., Audergon, J. M. (Eds.), Seminario Calidad Postcosecha y Productos Derivados en Frutos de Hueso, Universidad de Lleida, Spain 37-54.

Wang, H. and Ryser, E. T. (2014). Efficacy of various sanitizers against *Salmonella* during simulated commercial packing of tomatoes. *Journal of Food Protection*, *77*, 1868-1875.

Watada, A. E. and Qi, L. (1999). Quality of fresh-cut produce. *Postharvest Biology and Technology*, *15*, 201-205.

Wills, R. B. H., Mc Glasson, W. B., Graham, D. and Joyce, D. C. (2007). Postharvest. Anintroduction to the physiology and handling of fruit, vegetables and ornamentals. University of new South Wales Press Ltd. Australia, 29-50.

Yang, S. F. and Hoffman, N. E. (1984). Ethylene biosynthesis and its regulation in higher plants. *Annual Review of Plant Physiology*, *35*, 155-89.

Zhou, H. W., Lurie, S., Lers, A., Khatchitski, A., Sonego, L. and Ben Arie, R. (2000). Delayed storage and controlled atmosphere storage of nectarines: two strategies to prevent woolliness. *Postharvest Biology and Technology*, *18*, 133-141.

In: Apricots and Peaches
Editor: Jeanne Hansen

ISBN: 978-1-63484-684-4

Chapter 4

IMPACT OF HEAT PROCESSING ON NUTRITIONAL AND FUNCTIONAL PROPERTIES OF PEACH

Ana Oliveira and Manuela Pintado*

Centro de Biotecnologia e Química Fina – Laboratório Associado,
Escola Superior de Biotecnologia,
Universidade Católica Portuguesa/Porto, Porto, Portugal

ABSTRACT

Peach is a fruit with high content of phytochemical compounds with antioxidant activity, namely polyphenols and carotenes that make them a healthy fruit for consumers. Peach (*Prunus persica* (L.)), is an important commercial Mediterranean fruit during summer season not only for its high water content, fibre and minerals, but also for its high content in antioxidant molecules such as procyanidins, anthocyanins, catechins, phenolic acids and carotenoids (lutein, zeaxanthin, β-cryptoxanthin and β-carotene). These compounds in peach fruit vary strongly in relation to different environmental and agricultural factors, such as cultivar, rootstock, water and ripening stage at harvest.

Besides the regular peach consumption as fresh fruit, processed products such as juices, jams, jellies, smoothies, canned fruit and others, are usually produced from fruit fresh market.

* Corresponding author. Tel.: +351 225580097. E-mail address: mpintado@porto.ucp.pt (Manuela Pintado).

Information about nutrient content of processed fruits is of interest to consumers as they are becoming more aware and interested about their related health benefits. Fruit processing and storage may lead to negative or positive effects concerning their nutritional value according the processing steps they are exposed to. There are occurrences during fruit processing where chemical reactions could release bound components leading to a promotion of nutritional quality.

Among the phytochemicals, phenols, have received a great deal of attention because of their antioxidant activity, which help to neutralise free radicals. Thermal treatment is one of the most important factors affecting their stability. Previous studies have shown that concentrations of carotenoids often increase during heat treatment, probably because cell walls are softened, making the extraction of carotenoids easier during analysis. Extreme or prolonged heat treatment, however, enhances loss of carotenoids. Factors such as light, metals, oxygen, organic acids and heat can promote carotenoid isomerization and degradation.

The aim of this chapter, therefore, is to review the impact of different industrial processing techniques of sterilization and associated storage conditions (e.g., time and temperature) on nutritional and functional characteristics of processed peach, and to establish their role on the nutritional and functional quality of fruit.

1. Introduction

According to the World Health Organization – WHO, a healthy diet for adults should include at least 400 g (5 portions) of fruit and vegetables a day in order to reduce the risk of noncommunicable diseases (NCDs), including obesity, diabetes, heart disease, stroke and cancer and helps ensure an adequate daily intake of dietary fibre (WHO and Consultation, 1990). Due to these food-based dietary guidelines fruit and vegetable consumption is growing rapidly in recent years. Associated with the new consumer's profile and life style more convenient food products are required, and consequently there is an increasing demand for ready to eat products (Rickman, Barrett, and Bruhn, 2007).

For this reason, the market of processed fruits and vegetables has been growing in recent decades as a result of changes in consumer attitudes.

Peach is a fruit rich in phytochemical compounds with high antioxidant activity, mainly associated to polyphenols and carotenoids that make them a healthy fruit for consumers. Peach (*Prunus persica* (L.) Batsch), is an important commercial Mediterranean fruit during summer season not only for its high water content, fibre and minerals, but also for its richness in antioxidant molecules such as procyanidins, anthocyanins, catechins and phenolic acids, i.e., hydroxycinnamates (Tomás-Barberán et al., 2001) and carotenoids particularly lutein, zeaxanthin, β-cryptoxanthin and β-carotene (Dalla Valle, Mignani, Spinardi, Galvano, and Ciappellano, 2007). Asami, Hong, Barrett, and Mitchell (2003b) described peaches as a rich source of procyanidins with similar profiles to those found in cocoa, apples, wine and tea.

Several health benefits have been associated to the aforementioned antioxidant compounds. It has been proven that flavonoids (catechins, quercetins, proanthocyanidins) have protective effect against cardiovascular disease (Hertog et al., 1993; Hertog et al., 1995) and reduction of digestive tract cancer risk (Bushman, 1998).

Carotenoids, which are lipid soluble compounds, have been associated with protective effects against some types of cancer, age-related macular degeneration, and heart disease. Eye, skin and dental diseases have also been linked to decreased levels of dietary vitamin A precursors, which are usually obtained from carotenoids (Rojas-Garbanzo, Pérez, Bustos-Carmona and Vaillant, 2011).

The preventive role of carotenoids against disease has also been attributed to their strong antioxidant properties. They can capture oxygen free radicals (atoms or groups of atoms with an unshared electron) because of their conjugated double bonds system and the carotenoids with nine or more double bonds provide the highest protection (Rodriguez-Amaya, 1996).

As observed for other fruits, antioxidant compounds in peach fruit varies strongly in relation to different environmental and agricultural factors, such as cultivar (Cantin, Moreno and Gogorcena, 2009; Gil, Tomás-Barberán, Hess-Pierce and Kader, 2002; Tavarini, Degl'Innocenti, Remorini, Massai and Guidi, 2008), rootstock (Drogoudi and Tsipouridis, 2007; Giorgi et al., 2005; Remorini et al., 2008), water (Buendía, Allende, Nicolás, Alarcón and Gil, 2008) and ripening stage at harvest (Remorini et al., 2008). These conditions may lead to relevant variations on the type and content of these compounds present on commercial peaches.

Despites the high peach consumption as fresh fruit associated to its pleasant flavour and taste, they have a short shelf-life; for that reason a variety of processed products based on fresh fruit have been arising in the market juices, jams, jellies, smoothies, canned fruit and others, guaranteeing their presence throughout all the seasons (García-Parra et al., 2011). Carotenoids and other antioxidant compounds contribute to improve freshness and fruit products shelf-life used in industry (Hidalgo and Brandolini, 2008).

The bioacessibility of these compounds, whatever the source, is well known to be profoundly influenced by food processing (Hadley, Clinton and Schwartz, 2003). Previous studies have shown that concentrations of carotenoids often increase during heat treatment, probably because cell walls are softened, making the extraction of carotenoids easier during analysis (de Sá and Rodriguez-Amaya, 2003). Extreme or prolonged heat treatment, however, enhances loss of carotenoids. Factors such as light, metals, oxygen, organic acids and heat can promote carotenoid isomerization and degradation (Rodriguez-Amaya, 1996).

Information about nutrient content of processed fruits is of interest to consumers as they are becoming more aware and interested about their related health benefits. Fruit processing and storage may lead to detrimental or beneficial effects concerning their nutritional value according the processing steps they are exposed to. There are occurrences during fruit processing where chemical reactions could release bound components leading to an increase in nutritional quality (Ravichandran, Ahmed, Knorr and Smetanska, 2012), however, these processing techniques conditions can promote changes like cell wall and membrane disruption, enzyme catalysed conversion processes and chemical reactions that could affect phytochemicals richness of fruit (Patras, Brunton, O'Donnell and Tiwari, 2010).

2. Impact of Thermal Processing on Nutritional and Functional Properties of Peaches

In all its forms of application, thermal processing persists as the most widely used method of preserving and extending the useful shelf-life of foods. The concept of in-container sterilization involves the application of a high-temperature thermal treatment for a sufficiently long time to destroy microorganisms of public health and spoilage concerns (Pereira and Vicente, 2010). The hermetic seal maintains an environment in the container that prevents the growth of other microorganisms of higher resistance and most importantly, prevents pathogens from producing toxins during storage and eventual recontamination (Awuah, Ramaswamy and Economides, 2007).

Thermal processing of foods, which involves heating to temperatures ranging from 50 to 150°C (Patras et al., 2010), depends on factors such as (i) the physical characteristics of the food product including thermo-physical properties, shape and size of the container holding the product, (ii) the type and thermal resistance of the target microorganisms that are likely to be present in the food, and (iii) the pH, water activity (*a*w) and salt content of the food (Fellows, 2009).

The use of heat through thermal processing operations, which among others include pasteurization, sterilization, drying and evaporation, is still a common practice of food industries in order to guarantee the microbiological safety of their products as well as enzyme inactivation. These traditional heating methods rely essentially on the generation of heat outside the product to be heated, by combustion of fuels or by an electric resistive heater, and its transference into the product through conduction and convection mechanisms (Pereira and Vicente, 2010). Conventional heat treatments are prone to induce permanent changes to the nutritional, biochemical and sensory attributes of foods (Aguilar-Rosas, Ballinas-Casarrubias, Nevarez-Moorillon, Martin-Belloso and Ortega-Rivas, 2007). Therefore, recent developments in food processing operations have aimed at technologies that have the potential to substantially reduce damage to nutrients and sensory components by way of reduced heating times and optimized heating temperatures (Awuah et al., 2007).

Thermal treatments involves blanching (water, steam, vacuum-steam, in-can and hot-air) (Thane and Reddy, 1997); thermal drying (Prakash, Jha and Datta, 2004) such as sun drying, cross-flow, fluidized bed, osmotic air drying, oven drying, drum, spray, puff, freeze and microwave drying (Rawson et al., 2011).

Changes in processed products may be desirable; the rather harsh temperature for an extended period of time would trigger chemical reactions, and loss of nutrients and sensory characteristics such as appearance, colour, flavor and texture. Vitamins are among the most sensitive food components to be affected by heat sterilization (vitamins A, D, E), β-carotene, Vitamin C (ascorbic acid), Vitamins B1 (thiamine), B2 (riboflavin), nicotinic acid, pantothenic acid and biotin C (Ryley and Kajda, 1994).

Mild heat treatment can trigger Maillard reactions, which are a complex series of reactions between proteins and reducing sugars. The reaction is characterized by colourless solution, but after several reactions, brown or black insoluble compounds called melanoidins are formed (Awuah et al., 2007).

The nutritional value of the product will be compromised by protein damage and loss of amino acids, including lysine, L-arginine, and L-histidine.

Natural occurring pigments in foods are susceptible to changes or degradation by heat such as chlorophylls (in photosynthetic tissues), anthocyanins (the red and blue hues associated with many fruits and vegetables), carotenoids (found in fruits, dairy products, egg, fish and vegetables) and betanins (present in red beet roots and meat) influencing consumer acceptability (Awuah et al., 2007) and the nutritional value that has been ascribed to several of these compounds.

Peaches are commonly preserved by thermal processing methods such as canning. The thermal process applied to peaches is typically greater than that required for microbiological destruction in order to assist texture softening to a degree that the fruit is acceptable to the consumer. There have been few studies on the effect of processing on phenolic composition in peaches (Oliveira et al., 2016; Oliveira et al., 2015; Oliveira, Gomes, Alexandre, Almeida and Pintado, 2014; Oliveira, Pintado and Almeida, 2012), even though variations in phenolic composition have been shown to impact the antioxidant capacity of processed peaches (Asami et al., 2003b) (Table 1). Hernandez et al. (1997) reported a decrease in cinnamic acids and derivatives, flavonols and flavan-3-ols of peach juices with thermal treatment by microwave at 105ºC for 45 s or 120ºC for 20 min. Hong, Barrett, and Mitchell (2004) reported a reduction in the content of procyanidins when peach slices were canned at 104ºC for 10 min. These studies demonstrated that different processes gave rise to a series of changes in the phenolic composition and that flavan-3-ol monomers were not detected after the thermal treatments. Arts, van de Putte, and Hollman (2000) showed that a 19.7% loss in (+)-catechin occurred in canned peaches purchased at market. Talcott, Howard, and Brenes (2000) reported an increase in the content of some phenolics such as neochlorogenic and chlorogenic acids and decrease in (+)-catechin and caffeic acid on fresh peaches blanched for either a long (20 min) or short (2 min) time and after the maceration to purées, which were pasteurized in boiling water for 30 min. The increase of these compounds under pasteurization mainly in short blanched samples may provide evidence for reactions caused by either polymer formation or isomerization of the parent compound. García-Parra et al. (2011) studied the impact of thermal treatment (85ºC, 5 min) on peach purée and (Oliveira et al., 2012) studied on peach pieces. Both observed a higher stability in polyphenols, but some carotenoids have decreased such as zeaxanhin and β–cryptoxanthin as reported for peach pieces (Table 1). On contrary, Lavelli, Pompei, and Casadei (2008) reported a decrease on phytochemicals when peach purée was pasteurized at 100ºC for 5 min. Authors pointed out air incorporation in the pulping/finishing and the involvement of polyphenol oxidase (PPO) and peroxidase (POD) as the reasons for the lower content in antioxidant compounds.

Table 1. Effect of conventional thermal processing on peach bioactive compounds

Variety	Type	Conditions	Impact on the bioactive compounds	References
Not provided	Juice	Microwave at 105°C for 45 s or 120°C for 20 min	(↓) Chlorogenic acid (↓) p-Coumaric acid (↓) p-Coumaroylquinic acid (↓) (+)-Catechin	(Hernandez et al., 1997)
Not provided	Purée	Stem blanched for 2 and 20 min and pasteurized boiling water 30 min	(↑) Total phenolics (↑) Neochlorogenic acid (↑) Chlorogenic acid (↓) (+)-catechin (↓) Caffeic acid	(Talcott et al., 2000)
Batsch	Slices	Commercially Canned	(↓) (+)-Catechin	(Arts et al., 2000)
Ross	Slices	Canned at 104°C for 10 min and 110°C for 2.4 min	(↓) Total phenolics (↓) Procyanidins	(Asami, Hong, Barrett and Mitchell, 2003a; Asami et al., 2003b)
Ross	Slices	Canned at 104°C for 10 min	(↓) Procyanidins	(Hong et al., 2004)
Redhaven Elegant Lady	Purée	Pasteurized at 100°C, 5 min	(↓) Total phenolic (↓) Neochlorogenic acid (↓) Chlorogenic acid (↓) Procyanidins (↓) (+)-Catechin (↓) Quercetin-3-O-glucoside (↓) Cyanidin-3-glucoside (↓) β-carotene	(Lavelli et al., 2008)

Table 1. (Continued)

Variety	Type	Conditions	Impact on the bioactive compounds	References
Not provided	Purée	Pasteurized at 85°C, 5 min	(↔) Total antioxidant (↔) Total phenolic (↔) Total carotenoids (↔) β-carotene (↔) Zeaxanthin+Lutein	(García-Parra et al., 2011)
Catherine	Pieces	Pasteurized at 84.5°C, 5 min	(↓) Total antioxidant (↔) Total phenolic (↓) Total carotenoids (↓) Protocatechuic acid (↔) Catechin (↔) Epicatechin (↔) Rutin (↔) Chlorogenic acid (↔) Neochlorogenic acid (↓) Zeaxanthin (↓) β-Cryproxanthin (↔) β-Carotene (↔) Lutein	(Oliveira et al., 2012)

Where (↓) refers to decrease in the content, (↑) refers to increase in the content and (↔) refers to neither increase nor decrease in the content of bioactive compounds.

3. Novel Thermal Processing Techniques

As mentioned before, the use of heat through thermal processing operations is still a common practice of the food industries in order to guarantee the microbiological safety of their products. However, these ways of processing are still limited due to considerable losses of heat on the surfaces of the equipment and installations (Pereira and Vicente, 2010).

Quite recently, alternative or novel food processing methods (both thermal and non-thermal) have emerged and are being explored to produce safer and better quality foods. These alternative technologies which include but are not limited to: high-pressure processing, pulsed electric field, pulsed X-ray or ultraviolet light, ohmic heating, radio frequency, microwave, pulsed light, and oscillating magnetic fields that could potentially replace conventional thermal processes for some products. The food industry is actively involved in these developments, and poised to adopt new technological alternatives that offer competitive advantages (Awuah et al., 2007).

Ohmic heating and dielectric heating, which includes radio frequency (RF) and microwave (MW) heating, are promising alternatives to conventional methods of heat processing. In these novel thermal technologies energy is generated directly inside the food, allowing to reduce the excessive cooking times observed during conventional thermal treatments (Pereira and Vicente, 2010).

Irradiation is the process of applying low levels of radiant energy to a material to sterilize or preserve it. It is a physical means of food processing that involves exposing the prepackaged or bulk foodstuffs to gamma rays, x-rays, or electrons; foodstuffs using an electron accelerator (Mahapatra, Muthukumarappan and Julson, 2005).

The applications of microwave heating in food processing include drying, pasteurization, sterilization, thawing, tempering, baking of food materials. Microwave heating achieve high heating rates, significant reduction in cooking time, more uniform heating, safe handling, ease of operation and low maintenance (Chandrasekaran, Ramanathan and Basak, 2013; Salazar-González, San Martín-González, López-Malo and Sosa-Morales, 2012; M. Zhang, Tang, Mujumdar and Wang, 2006).

High hydrostatic pressure (HHP) is an easy industrialized non-thermal processing technology, in which a food is subjected to pressures up to 600±10 MPa for several minutes to inactivate microorganisms at temperatures less than 40°C (Bull et al., 2004). Some studies indicated that HHP was effective in maintaining the texture of fresh-cut fruits due to limited tissue damage and cell wall separation (Islam, Igura, Shimoda and Hayakawa, 2003; Trejo Araya et al., 2009; F. Zhang et al., 2012).

Little is known about the impact of those novel thermal technologies in peach phytochemicals. Louarme and Billaud (2012) reported a decrease in the ascorbic acid content of peach dice and on chunky fruit desserts with peach dice when treated with ohmic heating at a flow rate of 300 L/h, total period of 12.36 min and for initial temperature of 20ºC, ending with 105ºC and cool down until 40ºC. García-Parra, González-Cebrino, Delgado, Lozano, Hernández and Ramírez, 2011) reported an increased extraction of carotenoids (lutein+zeaxanthin, β-cryptoxanthin and β-carotene), polyphenols and total antioxidant activity from nectarines (*P. persica*) treated with high-pressure processing (450 or 600 MPa for 5 or 10 min). High hydrostatic pressure treatment of peach juice at 400–600 MPa and 25ºC for 5–25 min preserved more L-ascorbic acid than thermal treatment (Rao et al., 2013).

4. Storage Conditions after Processing

During shelf-life period, fruit is generally stored and exposed to conditions (temperature, atmosphere, light and time) that could affect phytochemicals stability and availability.

Storage time after processing is a key variable with enormous implications in supply-chain management. Time is a central variable requiring management in all kinetic processes and determining the final concentrations of nutritional and bioactive compounds in foods and beverages. During storage chemical reactions involving bioactive phytochemicals proceed at different rates depending on variables intrinsic to food matrices as well as on variables related to storage conditions (Nicoli, Anese and Parpinel, 1999).

A number of studies have reported the significance of long-term storage effects on the retention of bioactive compounds in the finished fruit products (Table 2).

On peaches Hong et al. (2004) reported a decrease in procyanidins after 3 months storage at room temperature of canned slices. There is a time-related loss in higher oligomers; the levels of monomers had decreased by 10%, dimers by 16%, trimers by 45%, and tetramers by 80%. Asami et al. (2003b) reported a 30-43% loss in total phenolics on canned slices after 6 months under room temperature. Campbell and Padilla-Zakour (2013) reported for canned peach slices, stored for 6 months at 20ºC, an almost completely degradation of zeaxanthin and 20 and 38% decrease of phenolics and carotenoids, respectively. They also reported higher decrease after 6 months for peeled peaches than unpeeled. Storage of canned fruit can induce degradation of phytochemicals by oxidation, since after thermal action they can be exposed to oxygen.

On purées Talcott et al. (2000) reported an increase of (+)-catechin, chlorogenic and neochlorogenic acid as a result of thermal processing and a slow decline during storage due to oxidative degradation. On contrary, levels of caffeic acid were lost during pasteurization, but increased slightly in response to chlorogenic acid hydrolysis during storage. García-Parra et al. (2011) described some stability on carotenoids when peach purée was thermally processed (85ºC, 5 min) and stored 60 d under refrigerated temperatures (5°C), however, total phenolics and total antioxidant capacity decreased.

Thermal treatment can increase the extractability of carotenoids. However, during storage the interaction between carotenoids and some food components such as the ascorbic acid added could have reduced carotene oxidation (Young and Lowe, 2001).

Table 2. Effect of storage after conventional thermal processing on peach bioactive compounds

Variety	Type	Conditions	Impact on the bioactive compounds	References
Ross	Slices	Canned and stored 3 months at room temperature	(↓) Procyanidins	(Hong et al., 2004)
Ross	Slices	Canned and stored 6 months at room temperature	(↓) Total phenolics	(Asami et al., 2003a, 2003b)
Not provided	Purée	Immersed boiling water 30 min and stored 4 weeks at 40°C	(↓) Total phenolic (↓) Neochlorogenic acid (↓) Chlorogenic acid (↑) Caffeic acid	(Talcott et al., 2000)
Redhaven Elegant Lady	Purée	12 months at 37°C	(↓) Total phenolic (↓) Neochlorogenic acid (↓) Chlorogenic acid (↓) Procyanidins (↓) (+)-Catechin (↓) Quercetin-3-O-glucoside (↓) Cyanidin-3-glucoside (↓) β-carotene	(Lavelli et al., 2008)
Elegant Lady Redhaven Springbelle	Nectars	3 months at 23 and 37°C	(↓) Total antioxidant capacity (↓) Neochlorogenic acid	(Lavelli, Pompei and Casadei, 2009)

Table 2. (Continued)

Variety	Type	Conditions	Impact on the bioactive compounds	References
			(↓) Chlorogenic acid (↓) (+)-Catechin (↓) Quercetin-3-O-glucoside (↔) β-carotene	
Not provided	Purée	60 d at 5ºC	(↓) Total antioxidant capacity (↓) Total phenolic (↔) Total carotenoids (↔) β-carotene (↔) Zeaxanthin+Lutein	(García-Parra et al., 2011)
John Boy II PF 23 Redhaven	Slices	Canned and stored 6 months at 20ºC	(↓) Total antioxidant capacity (↓) Total phenolic (↓) Total carotenoids (↓) β-carotene (↓) Zeaxanthin (↓) Flavonol glycosides	(Campbell and Padilla-Zakour, 2013)
Catherine	Pieces	Pasteurized at 84.5ºC, 5 min	(↓) Total antioxidant (↓) Total phenolic (↓) Total carotenoids (↓) Catechin (↓) Epicatechin (↓) Rutin (↑) Chlorogenic acid (↑) Neochlorogenic acid (↑) Zeaxanthin (↓) β-Cryproxanthin (↓) β-Carotene (↓) Lutein	(Oliveira et al., 2012)

Where (↓) refers to decrease in the content, (↑) refers to increase in the content and (↔) refers to neither increase nor decrease in the content of bioactive compounds.

On contrary, Lavelli et al. (2008) reported a decrease in β-carotene and phenolics on industrial processed purées stored 12 months at 37ºC after thermal treatment (100ºC, 5 min). However, peach nectars stored 3 months at 37ºC presented stability on β-carotene, but showed a decrease in the remaining polyphenols such as (+)-catechin, chlorogenic acid, neochlorogenic acid, etc. Also, an increase of storage temperature from 23 to 37ºC caused a 3.5 fold increase in the degradation rate constant (Table 2) for these compounds. Oliveira et al. (2012) reported a gradual dissociation during storage of zeaxanthin from the native protein complex stimulated by previous heat treatment (85ºC, 5 min) was the explanation given for the zeaxanthin increase in peach pieces after 3 months storage at room temperature. The authors also reported the effect of the heat-inactivation of polyphenoloxidase (PPO), which is an enzyme responsible for the conversion of chlorogenic and neochlorogenic acids into quinones, preserving their levels during storage.

CONCLUSION

Consumers continue to demand for natural, fresh, and minimally processed foods, while modern food distribution systems require an adequate shelf-life associated to more convenient products.

Traditional technologies used in thermal processing of peaches have proven to be effective in terms of product safety. High temperature treatments can affect levels of bioactive compounds such polyphenols and carotenoids thereby reducing the antioxidant activities in processed peach and derived products. The mechanisms by which bioactive compounds degrade are not well known. However, in some studies antioxidant activity increased after processing, which could be a result of thermal effect on physical properties of the fruit.

To ensure food safety and at the same time to meet the retention of bioactive compounds, the interest in novel thermal preservation techniques have increased. These technologies represent a rapid, efficient and reliable alternative to improve the quality of food, but it also has the potential to develop new products with a unique functionality. Polyphenols and carotenoids presented different behaviours, since in some cases increased as a result of the improved extraction and in another's situations decreased as a result of degradation reactions. Changes in polyphenols generated consequently modifications in antioxidant capacity, and even the intermediated compounds formed during degradation can exhibited higher scavenging capacity. Bioactive compounds continue changing during storage after thermal processing. Storage temperature is a determinant factor in chemical reactions occurring in the majority of the compounds. Matrix modifications during processing and subsequent storage can also affect carotenoids solubility leading to an increased extraction.

The need to optimize processes in terms of quality and operating costs while meeting all safety requirements, demand more research to better understanding the thermal and non-thermal effect on physicochemical mechanisms and on functional properties of peaches. In this sense, it will contribute to create alternatives to the existing technologies in the industry to generate more nutritious processed food products.

REFERENCES

Aguilar-Rosas, S. F., Ballinas-Casarrubias, M. L., Nevarez-Moorillon, G. V., Martin-Belloso, O. and Ortega-Rivas, E. (2007). Thermal and pulsed electric fields pasteurization of apple juice: Effects on physicochemical properties and flavour compounds. *Journal of Food Engineering,* 83(1), 41-46.

Arts, I. C. W., van de Putte, B. and Hollman, P. C. H. (2000). Catechin contents of foods commonly consumed in the Netherlands. 1. Fruits, vegetables, staple foods, and processed foods. *Journal of Agricultural and Food Chemistry,* 48(5), 1746-1751.

Asami, D. K., Hong, Y.-J., Barrett, D. M. and Mitchell, A. E. (2003a). Comparison of the Total Phenolic and Ascorbic Acid Content of Freeze-Dried and Air-Dried Marionberry, Strawberry, and Corn Grown Using Conventional, Organic, and Sustainable Agricultural Practices. *Journal of Agricultural and Food Chemistry,* 51(5), 1237-1241.

Asami, D. K., Hong, Y.-J., Barrett, D. M. and Mitchell, A. E. (2003b). Processing-induced changes in total phenolics and procyanidins in clingstone peaches. *Journal of the Science of Food and Agriculture*, 83(1), 56-63.

Awuah, G. B., Ramaswamy, H. S. and Economides, A. (2007). Thermal processing and quality: Principles and overview. Chemical Engineering and Processing: *Process Intensification*, 46(6), 584-602.

Buendía, B., Allende, A., Nicolás, E., Alarcón, J. J. and Gil, M. I. (2008). Effect of regulated deficit irrigation and crop load on the antioxidant compounds of peaches. *Journal of Agricultural and Food Chemistry,* 56(10), 3601-3608.

Bull, M. K., Zerdin, K., Howe, E., Goicoechea, D., Paramanandhan, P., Stockman, R., Sellahewa, J., Szabo, E. A., Johnson, R. L. and Stewart, C. M. (2004). The effect of high pressure processing on the microbial, physical and chemical properties of Valencia and Navel orange juice. *Innovative Food Science and Emerging Technologies*, 5(2), 135-149.

Bushman, J. L. (1998). Green tea and cancer in humans: a review of the literature. *Nutrition and Cancer,* 31(3), 151-159.

Campbell, O. E. and Padilla-Zakour, O. I. (2013). Phenolic and carotenoid composition of canned peaches (Prunus persica) and apricots (Prunus armeniaca) as affected by variety and peeling. *Food Research International,* 54(1), 448-455.

Cantin, C. M., Moreno, M. A. and Gogorcena, Y. (2009). Evaluation of the antioxidant capacity, phenolic compounds, and vitamin C content of different peach and nectarine [Prunus persica (L.) Batsch] breeding progenies. *Journal of Agricultural and Food Chemistry*, 57(11), 4586-4592.

Chandrasekaran, S., Ramanathan, S. and Basak, T. (2013). Microwave food processing—A review. *Food Research International,* 52(1), 243-261.

Dalla Valle, A., Mignani, I., Spinardi, A., Galvano, F. and Ciappellano, S. (2007). The antioxidant profile of three different peaches cultivars (Prunus persica) and their short-term effect on antioxidant status in human. *European Food Research and Technology,* 225(2), 167-172.

de Sá, M. C. and Rodriguez-Amaya, D. B. (2003). Carotenoid composition of cooked green vegetables from restaurants. *Food Chemistry*, 83(4), 595-600.

Drogoudi, P. D. and Tsipouridis, C. G. (2007). Effects of cultivar and rootstock on the antioxidant content and physical characters of clingstone peaches. *Scientia Horticulturae*, 115(1), 34-39.

Fellows, P. J. (2009). Food processing technology: principles and practice: *Elsevier.*

García-Parra, J., González-Cebrino, F., Delgado, J., Lozano, M., Hernández, T. and Ramírez, R. (2011). Effect of Thermal and High-Pressure Processing on the Nutritional Value and Quality Attributes of a Nectarine Purée with Industrial Origin during the Refrigerated Storage. *Journal of Food Science*, 76(4), C618-C625.

Gil, M. I., Tomás-Barberán, F. A., Hess-Pierce, B. and Kader, A. A. (2002). Antioxidant capacities, phenolic compounds, carotenoids, and vitamin C contents of nectarine, peach, and plum cultivars from California. Journal of Agricultural and Food Chemistry, 50(17), 4976-4982.

Giorgi, M., Capocasa, F., Scalzo, J., Murri, G., Battino, M. and Mezzetti, B. (2005). The rootstock effects on plant adaptability, production, fruit quality, and nutrition in the peach (cv.'Suncrest'). *Scientia Horticulturae,* 107(1), 36-42.

Hadley, C. W., Clinton, S. K. and Schwartz, S. J. (2003). The consumption of processed tomato products enhances plasma lycopene concentrations in association with a reduced lipoprotein sensitivity to oxidative damage. *The Journal of nutrition,* 133(3), 727-732.

Hernandez, T., Auśn, N., Bartolomé, B., Bengoechea, L., Estrella, I. and Gómez-Cordovés, C. (1997). Variations in the phenolic composition of fruit juices with different treatments. *Zeitschrift für Lebensmitteluntersuchung und-Forschung A,* 204(2), 151-155.

Hertog, M. G., Feskens, E. J., Kromhout, D., Hertog, M., Hollman, P. and Katan, M. (1993). Dietary antioxidant flavonoids and risk of coronary heart disease: the Zutphen Elderly Study. *The Lancet,* 342(8878), 1007-1011.

Hertog, M. G., Kromhout, D., Aravanis, C., Blackburn, H., Buzina, R., Fidanza, F., Giampaoli, S., Jansen, A., Menotti, A. and Nedeljkovic, S. (1995). Flavonoid intake and long-term risk of coronary heart disease and cancer in the seven countries study. *Archives of Internal Medicine,* 155(4), 381-386.

Hidalgo, A. and Brandolini, A. (2008). Kinetics of Carotenoids Degradation during the Storage of Einkorn (Triticum monococcum L. ssp. monococcum) and Bread Wheat (Triticum aestivum L. ssp. aestivum) Flours. *Journal of Agricultural and Food Chemistry,* 56(23), 11300-11305.

Hong, Y.-J., Barrett, D. M. and Mitchell, A. E. (2004). Liquid chromatography/mass spectrometry investigation of the impact of thermal processing and storage on peach procyanidins. *Journal of Agricultural and Food Chemistry,* 52(8), 2366-2371.

Islam, M. S., Igura, N., Shimoda, M. and Hayakawa, I. (2003). Effects of low hydrostatic pressure and moderate heat on texture, pectic substances and color of carrot. *European Food Research and Technology*, 217(1), 34-38.

Lavelli, V., Pompei, C. and Casadei, M. A. (2008). Optimization of colour and antioxidant activity of peach and nectarine puree: Scale-up study from pilot to industrial plant. *Journal of Agricultural and Food Chemistry*, 56(16), 7091-7099.

Lavelli, V., Pompei, C. and Casadei, M. A. (2009). Quality of nectarine and peach nectars as affected by lye-peeling and storage. *Food Chemistry,* 115(4), 1291-1298.

Louarme, L. and Billaud, C. (2012). Evaluation of ascorbic acid and sugar degradation products during fruit dessert processing under conventional or ohmic heating treatment. *LWT - Food Science and Technology,* 49(2), 184-187.

Mahapatra, A. K., Muthukumarappan, K. and Julson, J. L. (2005). Applications of Ozone, Bacteriocins and Irradiation in Food Processing: A Review. Crit *Rev Food Sci Nutr,* 45(6), 447-461.

Nicoli, M., Anese, M. and Parpinel, M. (1999). Influence of processing on the antioxidant properties of fruit and vegetables. *Trends in Food Science and Technology,* 10(3), 94-100.

Oliveira, A., Alexandre, E. M., Coelho, M., Barros, R. M., Almeida, D. P. and Pintado, M. (2016). Peach polyphenol and carotenoid content as affected by frozen storage and pasteurization. *LWT-Food Science and Technology,* 66, 361-368.

Oliveira, A., Coelho, M., Alexandre, E. M. C., Gomes, M. H., Almeida, D. P. F. and Pintado, M. (2015). Effect of modified atmosphere on phytochemical profile of pasteurized peach purées. *LWT - Food Science and Technology,* 64(2), 520-527.

Oliveira, A., Gomes, M. H., Alexandre, E. M., Almeida, D. P. and Pintado, M. E. (2014). Impact of pH on phytochemical profile of pasteurized peach purée during storage. *Journal of Agricultural and Food Chemistry.*

Oliveira, A., Pintado, M. and Almeida, D. P. (2012). Phytochemical composition and antioxidant activity of peach as affected by pasteurization and storage duration. *LWT-Food Science and Technology,* 49(2), 202-207.

Patras, A., Brunton, N. P., O'Donnell, C. and Tiwari, B. K. (2010). Effect of thermal processing on anthocyanin stability in foods; mechanisms and kinetics of degradation. *Trends in Food Science and Technology,* 21(1), 3-11.

Pereira, R. and Vicente, A. (2010). Environmental impact of novel thermal and non-thermal technologies in food processing. *Food Research International*, 43(7), 1936-1943.

Prakash, S., Jha, S. and Datta, N. (2004). Performance evaluation of blanched carrots dried by three different driers. *Journal of Food Engineering,* 62(3), 305-313.

Rao, L., Guo, X., Pang, X., Tan, X., Liao, X. and Wu, J. (2013). Enzyme Activity and Nutritional Quality of Peach (Prunus persica) Juice: Effect of

High Hydrostatic Pressure. *International Journal of Food Properties*, 17(6), 1406-1417.

Ravichandran, K., Ahmed, A. R., Knorr, D. and Smetanska, I. (2012). The effect of different processing methods on phenolic acid content and antioxidant activity of red beet. *Food Research International,* 48(1), 16-20.

Rawson, A., Patras, A., Tiwari, B. K., Noci, F., Koutchma, T. and Brunton, N. (2011). Effect of thermal and non thermal processing technologies on the bioactive content of exotic fruits and their products: Review of recent advances. *Food Research International,* 44(7), 1875-1887.

Remorini, D., Tavarini, S., Degl'Innocenti, E., Loreti, F., Massai, R. and Guidi, L. (2008). Effect of rootstocks and harvesting time on the nutritional quality of peel and flesh of peach fruits. *Food Chemistry*, 110(2), 361-367.

Rickman, J. C., Barrett, D. M. and Bruhn, C. M. (2007). Nutritional comparison of fresh, frozen and canned fruits and vegetables. Part 1. Vitamins C and B and phenolic compounds. *Journal of the Science of Food and Agriculture,* 87(6), 930-944.

Rodriguez-Amaya, D. B. (1996). Assessment of the provitamin A contents of foods—the Brazilian experience. *Journal of Food Composition and Analysis,* 9(3), 196-230.

Rojas-Garbanzo, C., Pérez, A. M., Bustos-Carmona, J. and Vaillant, F. (2011). Identification and quantification of carotenoids by HPLC-DAD during the process of peach palm (Bactris gasipaes H.B.K.) flour. *Food Research International,* 44(7), 2377-2384.

Ryley, J. and Kajda, P. (1994). Vitamins in thermal processing. *Food Chemistry,* 49(2), 119-129.

Salazar-González, C., San Martín-González, M. F., López-Malo, A. and Sosa-Morales, M. E. (2012). Recent studies related to microwave processing of fluid foods. *Food and Bioprocess Technology,* 5(1), 31-46.

Talcott, S. T., Howard, L. R. and Brenes, C. H. (2000). Contribution of Periderm Material and Blanching Time to the Quality of Pasteurized Peach Puree. *Journal of Agricultural and Food Chemistry*, 48(10), 4590-4596.

Tavarini, S., Degl'Innocenti, E., Remorini, D., Massai, R. and Guidi, L. (2008). Preliminary characterisation of peach cultivars for their antioxidant capacity. *International Journal of Food Science and Technology*, 43(5), 810-815.

Thane, C. and Reddy, S. (1997). Processing of fruit and vegetables: effect on carotenoids. *Nutrition and Food Science,* 97(2), 58-65.

Tomás-Barberán, F. A., Gil, M. I., Cremin, P., Waterhouse, A. L., Hess-Pierce, B. and Kader, A. A. (2001). HPLC–DAD–ESIMS Analysis of Phenolic Compounds in Nectarines, Peaches, and Plums. *Journal of Agricultural and Food Chemistry*, 49(10), 4748-4760.

Trejo Araya, X. I., Smale, N., Zabaras, D., Winley, E., Forde, C., Stewart, C. M. and Mawson, A. J. (2009). Sensory perception and quality attributes of high pressure processed carrots in comparison to raw, sous-vide and cooked carrots. *Innovative Food Science and Emerging Technologies*, 10(4), 420-433.

WHO, J. and Consultation, F. E. (1990). Diet, nutrition and the prevention of chronic diseases: World Health Organization Geneva.

Young, A. J. and Lowe, G. M. (2001). Antioxidant and prooxidant properties of carotenoids. *Archives of Biochemistry and Biophysics,* 385(1), 20-27.

Zhang, F., Dong, P., Feng, L., Chen, F., Wu, J., Liao, X. and Hu, X. (2012). Textural Changes of Yellow Peach in Pouches Processed by High Hydrostatic Pressure and Thermal Processing During Storage. *Food and Bioprocess Technology,* 5(8), 3170-3180.

Zhang, M., Tang, J., Mujumdar, A. and Wang, S. (2006). Trends in microwave-related drying of fruits and vegetables. *Trends in Food Science and Technology,* 17(10), 524-534.

In: Apricots and Peaches
Editor: Jeanne Hansen

ISBN: 978-1-63484-684-4

Chapter 5

PHYSICO-CHEMICAL AND SENSORY CHARACTERIZATION OF *PESCABIVONA P.G.I.*, A SICILIAN WHITE FLESH PEACH CULTIVAR [*PRUNUS PERSICA* (L.) BATSCH]: A CASE STUDY

Giuseppe Montevecchi[1,*], Maria Gabriella Mellano[2,3], Giuseppe Vasile Simone[1], Francesca Masino[1,4], Cristina Bignami[1,4] and Andrea Antonelli[1,4]

[1]Centro di Ricerca Interdipartimentale per il Miglioramento e la Valorizzazione delle Risorse Biologiche Agro-Alimentari BIOGEST-SITEIA, Università degli Studi di Modena e Reggio Emilia, Tecnopolo di Reggio Emilia, Reggio Emilia, Italy

[2]Organizzazione Nazionale Assaggiatori Frutta (O.N.A.Frut.), Cuneo, Italy

[3]Dipartimento di Scienze Agrarie Forestali e Alimentari, Università degli Studi di Torino, Grugliasco, TO, Italy

[4]Dipartimento di Scienze della Vita (Area Scienze Agro-Alimentari), Università degli Studi di Modena e Reggio Emilia, Reggio Emilia, Italy

[*] Tel: +39-0522-523541, Fax: +39-0522-522027; Email: giuseppe.montevecchi@unimore.it

ABSTRACT

Pescabivona [*Prunus persica* (L.) Batch] is the name of an autochthonous peach population of the Middle-West of Sicily. Samples of the four *Pescabivona* landraces (*Murtiddara*, *Bianca*, *Agostina*, and *Settembrina*) were harvested at three different altitudes and analysed for chemical, physico-chemical, and sensory descriptors. The data obtained have supported the application for registration of *Pescabivona* as Protected Geographical Indication (P.G.I.).

Statistic data processing outlined a substantial match in the composition of the four landraces at the different altitudes, highlighting high values of flesh firmness corresponding to balanced sugar/acidity ratios, in particular for the late ripening landraces (*Agostina* and *Settembrina*). In addition, a large content of lactones (the key odorant molecules) was found. A good agreement between sensory evaluation and composition was observed. In particular, the sensory liking was correlated with the main ripeness parameters, as well as with the pulp firmness.

Therefore, in periods of the year when the quality of the peaches is generally decreasing, the chance of tasting firm fruits at physiological ripeness and with a pleasant sensory profile as showed by *Pescabivona* is not very common.

1. INTRODUCTION

The peach tree is native of China. Since the days of ancient Rome it found ideal conditions for adaptability in the Mediterranean area and from here it spread to Europe and then to America, as well.

In the Italian area, the breeding of peach varieties began in the late 1500s in Tuscany, but the genetic improvement started in 1900, only, when thousands of varieties were made up in order to extend the time of ripening and to lower the chilling requirement. The availability of cultivars that differ in chilling requirement from high to very low was crucial to extend the peach culture in new areas, such as Canada and subtropical zones (Liverani, 2008). Since the early 1950s, Italian peach culture was considered a model for European, North African, and Middle Eastern countries. The innovations adopted in Italy, such as techniques of agronomic management, novel forms of breeding and selection, and use of new rootstocks and cultivars (cvs.) boosted the evolution of modern European peach culture (Fideghelli, 2008). The sensory characteristics become interesting for breeders only in recent years (Liverani, 2008).

The Italian peach presented the highest production in Europe with an average of about 1.6 millions t/year (Bassi and Foschi, 2013). In Italy, the amount of peaches produced is second only to apples, although their market value is equivalent and peaches have a larger production area. In recent years, however, there is a decrease of new orchards and, to a greater extent, a reduction of the production (Fideghelli, 2012). This phenomenon mostly occurs in the regions with the highest production, such as Emilia Romagna and Campania, which precede Piedmont, Basilicata, Sicily, and Calabria (Fideghelli, 2012).

1.1. Botanical Traits

Peach tree [*Prunus persica* (L.) Batch] belongs to the *Rosaceae* family, subgenus *Amygdalus*, section *Euamygdalus*. It is a medium-sized plant (up to 8 m, averaging 4-6 m). The leaves are lance-shaped, with crenate or dentate margin. The flowers are hermaphrodite, commonly consisting of five petals with colour variable from white to dark red. The species is self-fertile, entomophilous and the pollination usually occurs with high rates of fertilization. The fruit set is usually abundant. The thinning is practiced to allow reaching suitable fruit size for marketing. The flowering time depends on the chilling units (CU) necessary to meet the needs of each cv., as well as the accumulation of heat units (growing degree hours: GDH). Depending on the requirements in cold, peach cvs. can be divided into subject to dormancy and evergreen (not subject to dormancy). These latters have continuous growth and are typical of tropical or subtropical climate, where they can fructify twice a year.

The cvs. that are subject to dormancy can be themselves divided into three bands of chilling requirement, with intermediate variations: very low (CU < 50), very high (CU > 1500), and medium (699 < CU < 900), like most of the commercial cvs.

1.2. General Fruit Description

The ripening period is more related to the cvs. than to the flowering time: the fruits can take from 55 to 270 days to ripen (depending on the cv.). The ripe fruit detaches for natural abscission from the peduncle that remains attached to the branch.

The fruit is a drupe, usually globular or elongated. There is also a fruit with flattened shape and small kernel. Although this latter is a genetically dominant character, the cvs. that produce these fruits did not found great appreciation by the consumers because of some specific fruit defects. Exception are Spain, where flat peaches now represent 14% of total marketed production (Iglesias, 2013) and Italy, where they are coming from the traditional local markets of Sicily to many other regions. The interest is confirmed by the increasing number of improved cultivars released since 2000 (Giovannini and Liverani, 2014).

The fruit weight varies from less than 50 g of wild plant peaches, to 80-110 g of the fruits of early ripening cvs., to about 700 g of selected cvs. The pulp can be adherent to the wooden kernel (clingstone or 'non-*spicche*' cvs.) or not ('*spicche*' cvs.), and the weight of kernel accounts for 5-8% of the whole fruit weight.

The thin skin that can be more or less adherent to the flesh is normally fuzzy, while the smooth skin, typical of nectarines, is due to a mutation that occurred in China and imported to Europe in the fourteenth century (Bassi and Piagnani, 2008). The skin colour ranges from white green to yellow up to carmine. The white and yellow skin ground colour and flesh colour are fruit traits of reference for pomological and commercial classification of peach cvs. The red over colour of the skin depends on the synthesis of anthocyanins. These red pigments may be present in the flesh, where they are generally located under the skin and close to the pit. Anthocyanins are not present in the flesh of the best cultivars of '*percoche*' since these pigments would be subject to browning during canning.

The pulpy, juicy, and sweet mesocarp can be yellow or white and this is the most common descriptor for classifying commercial cvs. (white peaches or yellow peaches). Both types can be associated with "red pulp" (Mendelian dominant), characterised by an abundant accumulation of anthocyanins. Sometimes the "blood" peaches and nectarines are considered for market differentiation, but currently, this particular trait does not have any commercial importance, except in local markets.

The phenotype allows to distinguish the different types of peaches, according to pulp texture: melting (M) fruits with soft pulp, non-melting (NM) fruits that maintain a firm texture even at full maturity, commonly used to be put in syrup, except in Spain, South Italy, Central and South America where they are also consumed fresh, and stony hard (SH) fruits that do not produce ethylene and remain very compact and crispy even in full maturity. Cvs. for fresh consumption usually belong to type M, although some NM fruits are appreciated by consumers, as well. However, there is great difference of speed and way of softening that makes difficult to exactly distinguish the different types (Bassi and Piagnani, 2008).

The taste traits are strongly affected by the amount and kind of sugars and organic acids present in the pulp and by their relative relationship (soluble solid content to titratable acidity ratio). The acidity allows the discrimination into "sub-acid" (pH > 4.0) and "normal acid" (pH < 3.9) fruit. At the same sugar content, "sub-acid" peaches result in sweeter fruits than "normal acid" ones (Bassi and Piagnani, 2008).

Finally, peaches taste is markedly affected by the flavour, as well (Bassi and Piagnani, 2008).

1.3. Sensory Analysis of Peaches: Overview

The peach has such a remarkable richness of taste, juiciness, and flavour that concur to become one of the most appreciated fruits by the consumers. Moreover, the wide range of peach varieties can really satisfy a very large number of consumers.

The sensory aspects are well differentiated among all groups of varieties: the nectarines are crisp, the peaches have a melting and juicy pulp, and the "*percoche*" have an important aromatic component. In addition, the white flesh fruits are very aromatic and the yellow flesh ones show a more delicate aroma. Generally speaking, the aroma of a peach is defined by the presence of lactones, which are perceived by the olfactory epithelium even at very low concentrations, and other compounds (aldehydes, aliphatic alcohols, esters, and terpenoids), each one with a well-defined scent. All these molecules are present in different concentrations for different parts of the fruit (epicarp, pulp, part near the core, apical or distal part of the fruit). During a sensory analysis test, it is therefore essential to be very careful in the preparation of the sample to be submitted to the panel of judges, so that it was actually representative of the whole fruit.

The content and the ratio of the different aromatic substances uniquely characterise each fruit and can become a requisite for the varietal identification and characterisation.

During ripening, the flavour profile of the peach is constantly changing, so it also provides information regarding the suitability of agricultural techniques, production, and commercial management.

As already described for the relationship between sugars and acids, it is possible to distinguish among balanced, acidic, or sub-acid fruits. These characteristics are due to genetic traits and production methods. They can be quantified by sensory analysis carried out by trained judges. According to the conditions of production and storage, the results may define a sensory profile for each cv., characterised by peculiar sensory traits (Pedrieri and Rapparini, 2008).

1.4. Nutritional Value

The general nutritional composition of the peach, the low fat content (0.1%), and the energy value of approximately 30 kcal/100 g makes this fruit useful in diets aimed at weight control. In fact, water represents about 90% of the pulp content. This makes the peach a good help against the dehydration.

Although the mineral salts represent only 0.3% of the fruit weight, they are so important during summertime when the temperature and the damp favour the perspiration and the loss of mineral elements that should be properly recovered. In 100 g of pulp, there is potassium (260 mg), followed by phosphorus (20 mg), magnesium (9 mg), calcium (8 mg), sodium (3 mg), iron (0.4 mg), zinc (0.35 mg), and copper (0.04 mg).

The simple sugars, mainly sucrose followed by fructose and glucose, represent about 6% of the peach weight (Esti et al., 1997). As soon as the sugars are absorbed, they are quickly turned into energy because of their crucial role in the metabolism of cerebral and blood cells.

The main organic acids, such as malic, citric, quinic, and succinic, constituted about 0.7% of the peach weight and contribute to define the general taste of the fruit. They have effect on the blood acid-base equilibrium and on the kind of microorganisms that compose the intestinal bacterial flora.

The average protein content is about 8% of the peach weight.

The peel corresponds at most at the 10% of the fruit weight (Cannella, 2008). It mainly consists of insoluble fibre that does not have any nutritional value, but it is important because favours the bowel movement. The soluble fibre represents the 50% of the total fibre that is about 1.6% of the peach weight. This fibre is mainly constituted by pectin that may concur to modulate the absorption of glucose and the consequent glycaemic peak.

Some components present in lower amount give peaches nutritional properties and also nutraceutical value. Despite the differences in antioxidant content due to the genetic traits of the cvs. (Tavarini et al., 2008), each peach supplies the body with about 10% of the daily requirement of vitamin C (L-ascorbic acid), the main antioxidant hydrophilic vitamin. Moreover, the peach contains other phytochemicals mainly active towards the defence from oxidising agents, such as β-carotene and xanthophylls (vitamin A precursors) that give the yellow flesh colour and are present only in small amount in white peaches, and polyphenols (Cannella, 2008; Layne and Bassi, 2008). It should be stressed that only the consumption of fresh peaches provides the highest healthy proprieties of phytochemicals. Phytochemicals can act in synergy with vitamins, fibres, and mineral salts to develop protective activity according to different biochemical mechanisms (induction of enzymes biosynthesis, inhibition of the formation of harmful molecules, dilution and neutralisation of carcinogenic substances, enhancing of the antioxidant activity of vitamins).

Even if the products of peach processing do not have the same healthy properties of the fresh fruit, nevertheless suitable productive lines can help preserving such characteristics. Moreover, the availability of early- and late-ripening cvs. allows the consume of fresh fruits for a long period of the year.

1.5. Breeding and Biodiversity

During the time, the "modern" yellow flesh cvs. widely replaced the "old" white flesh varieties. Although the old varieties were more appreciated for their sensory characteristics, nowadays the modern cvs. better meet the current commercial and productive needs (Liverani et al., 2006). In the last few years, however, breeding programs were developed to select fruits with features suitable for the market and to valorise again the white flesh peaches (Liverani et al., 2006; Bassi et al., 2010a; Bassi et al., 2010b; Bassi and Foschi, 2011).

Biodiversity offers many examples of local varieties with specific traits consistent with the production and commercial trends. Often, local varieties are limited to regional market for reasons not dependent on their quality characteristics. Among these varieties, *Pescabivona* is a white flesh peach that has a deep connection with its autochthonous territory that is located southwest of *Sicani* Mountains (Sicily), in the areas of the municipality of Bivona and neighbouring towns (Figure 1).

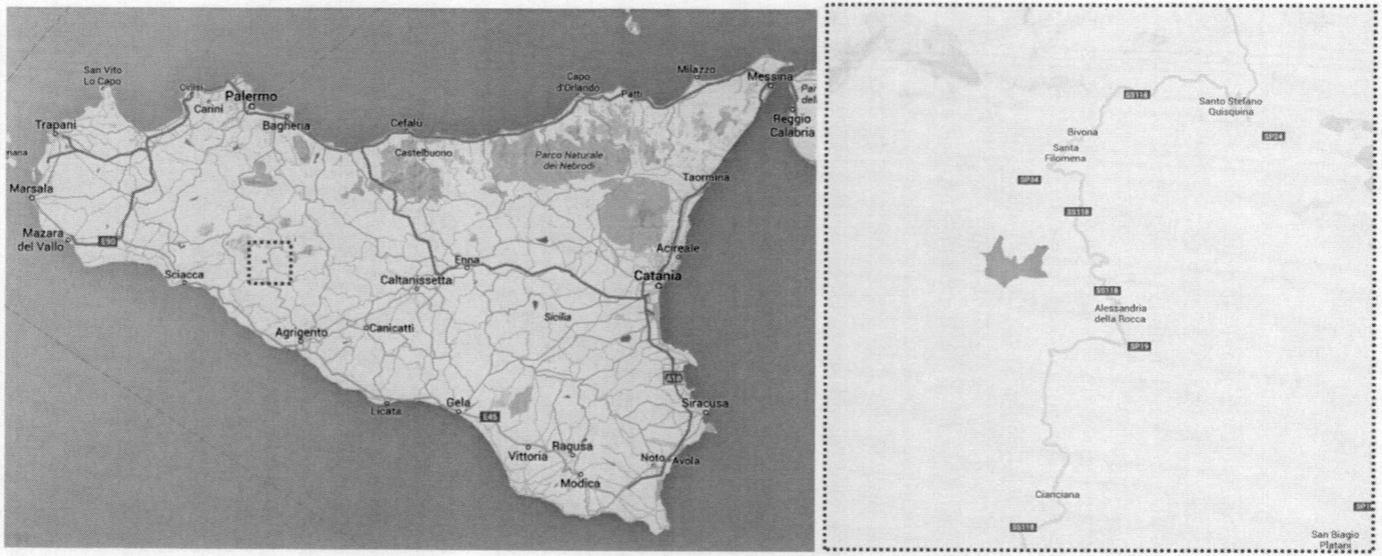

Figure 1. Graphical representation of the production area of *Pescabivona* (adapted from Vasile Simone et al., 2014).

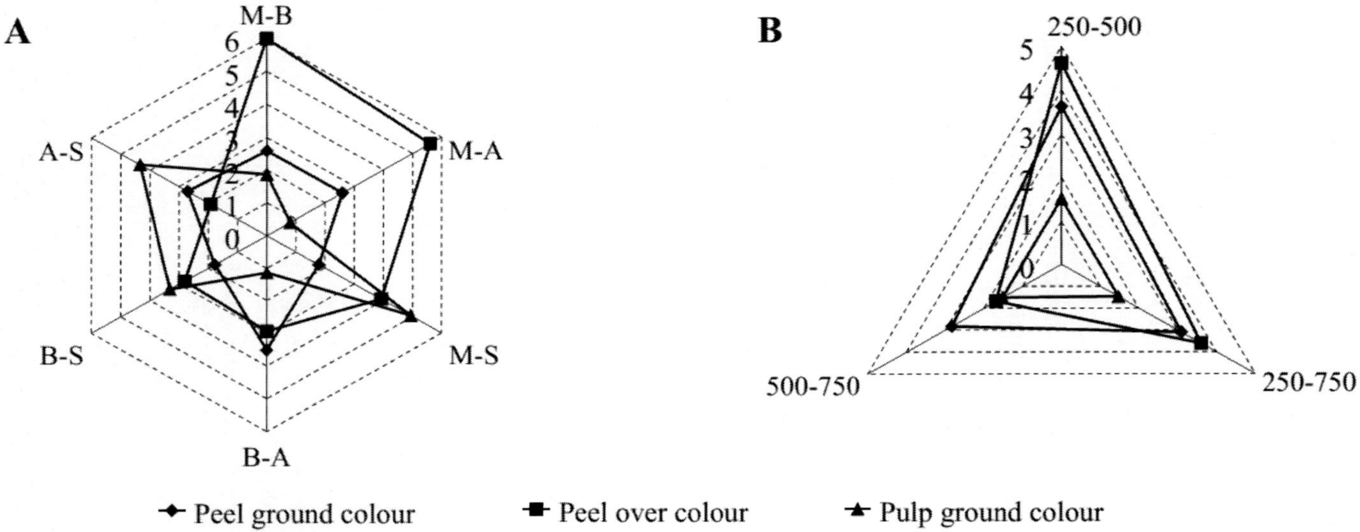

Figure 2. Colour distance related to peel ground colour, peel over colour, and pulp ground colour among landraces [A] and among altitudes [B]. *Murtiddara* (M), *Bianca* (B), *Agostina* (A), *Settembrina* (S) (from Montevecchi et al., 2012).

1.5.1. Pescabivona General Description and Aim of the Study

Pescabivona is a common name that indicates four landraces of autochthonous white flesh *Prunus persica* (L.) Batsch (Cusumano, 2009), originated by environmental and human selection (Marchese et al., 2006). The fruits are very appreciated by consumers for their sensory characteristics (Caruso et al., 2005). The first two landraces were identified and selected by local farmers around 1950 and named *Agostina* (Caruso, 1982) and *Settembrina*. They are both late ripening (late August and late September, respectively). With the spread of peach orchards in less mountainous areas, other two landraces were selected during the '70s. One with intermediate maturity (July) called *Bianca* and the last one that is early ripening (June) and called *Murtiddara* or *Primizia Bianca*.

This research aimed at showing the peculiar characteristics of *Pescabivona* fruits in order to confirm its quality even by comparison with the most common cvs. that are similar for type and ripening period.

These data provide information on the chemical, physico-chemical, and sensory characteristics of the fruits. This information is useful to all levels of the supply chain. In addition, the data obtained by the study represented a fundamental support to apply for "Protected Geographical Indication" (P.G.I.) recognition of *Pescabivona*. The favourable judgment for P.G.I. recognition was expressed by the Italian Ministry of Agriculture, Food and Forestry Policies (MiPAAF; G.U.R.I., n. 125 of 05/30/2013) and by the European Commission (O.J.E.U., C 103/13 of 8/4/2014).

2. Materials and Methods

2.1. Peach Sampling

Samples of the four *Pescabivona* peach landraces (*Murtiddara*, *Bianca*, *Agostina*, and *Settembrina*) were collected inside the growing area around Bivona (Sicily, Italy, lat. 37.619, long. 13.438) during all the harvest season.

Commercial orchards representative of the prevailing environmental, agronomic, and management conditions were identified. The orchards were grown on hilly-mountainous areas and exposed to the South. The soil was of a medium clay texture, with subalkaline reaction and normal quantities of macro and micronutrients. The plants were grafted on GF 677 or MRS 2/5 rootstocks, trained to vase and spaced 4 m × 4 m apart. Pruning, soil management, pest, and disease control were carried out according to the local traditional systems. Localized irrigation was supplied in the summer (Cusumano, 2009).

Sampling was carried out according to the following design. Since peach cultivation spans in Bivona from 250 to 750 m of altitude, the area was divided into three levels (250, 500, and 750 m a.s.l.), and a gross sample of 18 peaches was collected for each level and landrace by different trees. Each gross sample was portioned in three lots (6 peaches each) to have enough samples to carry out the analysis in triplicate (4 landraces × 3 altitudes × 3 replications = 36 samples).

The peaches were collected at "ready-to-eat" ripening stage evaluated by means of change in ground colour from green to yellow and fruit size corresponding to AA calibre (diameter from 73 to 80 mm, and circumference from 23 to 25 cm). Since peach quality shows variability within tree (Génard and Bruchou, 1992), fruit sampling was standardized under the following condition: middle vigour trees, rootstock GF 677, south exposure, external part of the canopy.

2.2. Reagents

Organic acids (citric, malic, quinic, and succinic acid), fructose, glucose, sucrose, (+)-catechin, chlorogenic acid, vitamin C, 2,2′-azino-bis(3-ethylbenzothiazoline-6-sulfonic acid) (ABTS), potassium persulphate, lactones (γ-decalactone, δ-decalactone, γ-dodecalactone, δ-dodecalactone), 2-octanol, *n*-undecane, and silica gel 100 C_{18} (particle size: 0.040–0.063 mm, not endcapped), were purchased from Fluka Sigma-Aldrich® (Milan, Italy). High purity solvents (acetonitrile, dichloromethane, ethanol, and methanol) were supplied by VWR International S.r.l. (Milan, Italy), while sulphuric and hydrochloric acids, and sodium hydroxide were purchased from Carlo Erba Reagents S.p.A. (Rodano, Milan, Italy). Deionized water was obtained by a Milli-Q purification system (Millipore, Milan, Italy).

2.3. Chemical and Physico-Chemical Determinations

The chemical and physico-chemical analysis were carried out at the laboratory of the Department of Life Sciences (Area Agro-Food Sciences) of the University of Modena and Reggio Emilia using the methods set up and described by Montevecchi and coll. (2012). Flesh colour, peel colour and over colour, colour distance, red percentage of the peel, weight, pulp firmness, pH, soluble solids content (SSC), titratable acidity (TA), SSC/TA ratio, main sugars and organic acids, aroma impact compounds (lactones), phenolics, and antioxidant capacity were the parameters evaluated.

The measure of colour was performed with a tristimulus reflectance colorimeter (Chroma meter CR-400, Konica Minolta) by detecting the coordinates L* (brightness), a*, and b* (colour components), C* (chroma), h (hue) of flesh, peel, and over colour of the peel. The coordinates were used to calculate the "colour distance" among landraces and between different altitudes (Billmeyer and Saltzman, 1981). The consistency of the pulp was measured with a Magness-Taylor-type penetrometer (MT) provided with a cylindrical metal probe (8 mm in diameter). The SSC was determined by a manual refractometer and TA by acid-base titration.

The values of the main ripeness and quality indexes were compared with those of the most widespread peach cvs. that are similar for category and time of harvest.

The determination of the analytes of interest was performed after extraction of the pulp in ethanol, following the method indicated by Pérez et al. (1997). By the same method, extracts of the peels were prepared in methanol for the determination of phenolic compounds and antioxidant activity.

Organic acids and sugars were identified and quantified according to the methods proposed by Chinnici and coll. (2005), with minor adjustments of the chromatographic conditions (Montevecchi et al., 2012). The ethanolic extracts were subjected to solid phase extraction (SPE cartridges, Isolute® SAX; Biotage, Uppsala, Sweden), followed by identification and quantification by HPLC. For sugars, a refractive index (RI) detector was used, while it was used an UV/Vis detector for organic acid determination (reading at 210 nm). The compounds of aroma impact were adsorbed on the solid phase (silica gel 100 C_{18}) dispersed directly in the hydroalcoholic extract (d-SPE technique); the separation and quantification were performed by GC-FID, and for each compound was calculated the odour activity value (Montevecchi et al., 2012).

Phenolics (total flavan-3-ols, read at 280 nm, and total hydroxycinnamic acids, read at 320 nm) were determined by a direct spectrophotometric reading and the results were expressed, respectively, as catechin and chlorogenic acid (Montevecchi et al., 2012). Finally, the antioxidant activity was measured according to the ABTS method (Re et al., 1999) and the results were expressed as mg vitamin C equivalent antioxidant capacity (VCEAC) per kg of fresh peach.

2.4. Sensory Analysis

Sensory analysis was carried out by *Organizzazione Nazionale Assaggiatori di Frutta* (O.N.A.Frut.) based in Cuneo (Italy), using the methods described in Montevecchi and coll. (2013). The four landraces were evaluated by a panel of trained judges in four different sessions, using a quantitative descriptive analysis by recording the intensity of each attribute on a 10-cm structured line scale anchored at each end. A few minutes before starting the session, the samples were prepared and presented to the judges peeled and cut into slices and gently stirred to reduce the variability. Nine sensory attributes related to colour, texture, odour, (retronasal) aroma, and taste of the analysed samples were evaluated: presence/absence of red veins near the stone, fibrousness, hardness, juiciness, intensity of smell, sweetness, sourness, bitterness, and aroma. Finally, each panelist was asked to express the overall liking to provide the potential consumer acceptance.

A descriptive evaluation of the whole fruit was carried out at the end of each panel session. Judges were asked to evaluate the geometric shape, symmetry of shape, peel ground colour, percentage and kind of peel blush colour, and intensity of smell.

2.5. Statistical Analysis

Statistical analyses (Analysis of variance – ANOVA, Tukey's multiple comparison test, linear regression analysis and principal component analysis – PCA) were carried out by means of the Statistica version 8.0 software (Stat Soft, Inc., Tulsa, U.S.A.).

3. Results and Discussion

3.1. Physical, Chemical and Physico-Chemical Determinations

3.1.1. Colour Parameters Measurement

The measurement of colour is an index of great importance in consumers' preferences (Infante et al., 2008). On a general level, a high homogeneity among samples was observed. In fact, statistically significant differences

($p \leq 0.05$) were observed only for pulp ground colour L* among landraces (Vasile Simone, 2014).

The most remarkable differences in the peel ground colour distance (Figure 2) were found by the comparison between *Bianca* and *Agostina*, while *Murtiddara-Settembrina* and *Bianca-Settembrina* resulted in the lowest colour distances (Montevecchi et al., 2012; Vasile Simone et al., 2014). The data for peel over colour distance allowed to classify *Murtiddara* apart from the other landraces, which showed a high homogeneity. Finally, *Settembrina* showed the highest distances in terms of pulp ground colour in comparison with all the other landraces that had shorter colour distance.

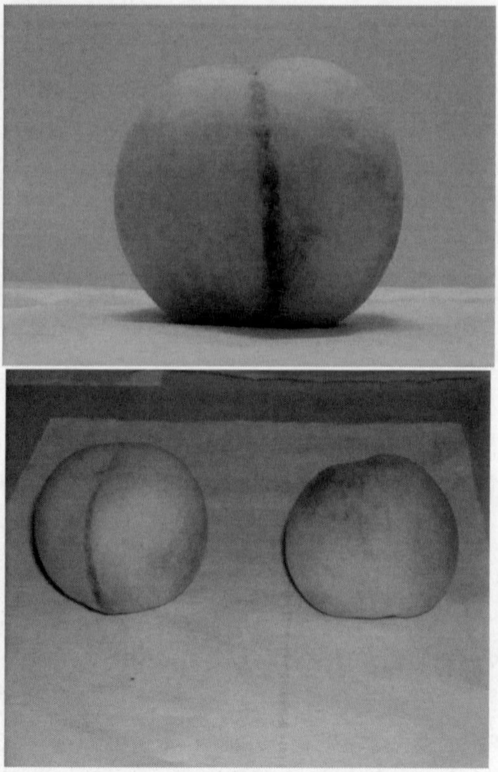

Figure 3. *Settembrina* with its typical red stripe along the suture line.

Peel over colour and peel ground colour for fruits grown at highest altitudes (500 and 750 m a.s.l.) showed higher homogeneity in comparison with fruits grown at 250 m a.s.l. (Figure 2). Conversely, pulp ground colour did not show similar discrepancies. Ultimately, considering the limited differences, the data indicated a substantial homogeneity of the fruits of the four landraces. The percentage of red of the peel, as well, did not show statistically significant differences, with all average values below 50% among the landraces (Montevecchi et al., 2012; Vasile Simone et al., 2014). Although there is currently a preference towards fruits with high amount of peel over colour, consumers' choices seem to be more influenced by the intensity of the yellow of the peel ground colour rather than the percentage of red (Liverani et al., 2008). *Settembrina* presents a characteristic red stripe (Figure 3) along the suture line, possibly due to mutations of the epidermis layer (Marchese et al., 2006).

3.1.2. Physico-Chemical Parameters

The pulp firmness showed growing values, in a quite regular way, among landraces during the progress of the harvest season (Figure 4). The lowest values were observed for *Murtiddara*, while the late ripening landraces, *Agostina* and *Settembrina*, showed the highest values. As reported by Cantín and coll. (2010), the average values found for pulp firmness, in particular for late ripening landraces, are typical of 'ready for market' fruits. Conversely, the values of SSC (expressed in °Bx) found in the samples are characteristic of 'ready-to-eat' fruits, as requested by the consumers' orientation (Liverani et al., 2008) (Figure 4). Pulp firmness is highly appreciated by consumers and correlated to the freshness and genuineness of fruits (Infante et al., 2008).

pH and TA allowed to classify the fruits as 'acids' (Dirlewanger et al., 1999), except *Agostina* that showed values of TA a little lower (Figure 4). On the other hand, the combination of SSC and TA is typical of fruits with a sweet taste (Bassi and Foschi, 2013). No statistically significant differences were showed for these three parameters among the different landraces and altitudes (Montevecchi et al., 2012; Vasile Simone et al., 2014). The ratio between soluble solid content and titratable acidity (SSC/TA), also known as ripening index (Cantín et al., 2010), provides a better evaluation on fruit sweetness (Infante et al., 2008). In fact, there is a negative correlation between acidity and sweetness: the higher the acidity the lower the perception of sweet taste. On the other hand, the perception of sweetness increases with °Bx, being constant the acidity (Castellari, 2002). SSC/TA showed relatively high values for the four landraces at all altitudes (ranged from 19.65 to 26.79), except *Murtiddara* 750 m a.s.l. This is probably due to the early harvest period (June) along with the high altitude. In particular, *Agostina* provided suitable results for all the altitudes. Generally speaking, all these parameters related to the sweetness and acidity showed very limited differences between the landraces, showing a higher variability among the areas of production within the same landrace.

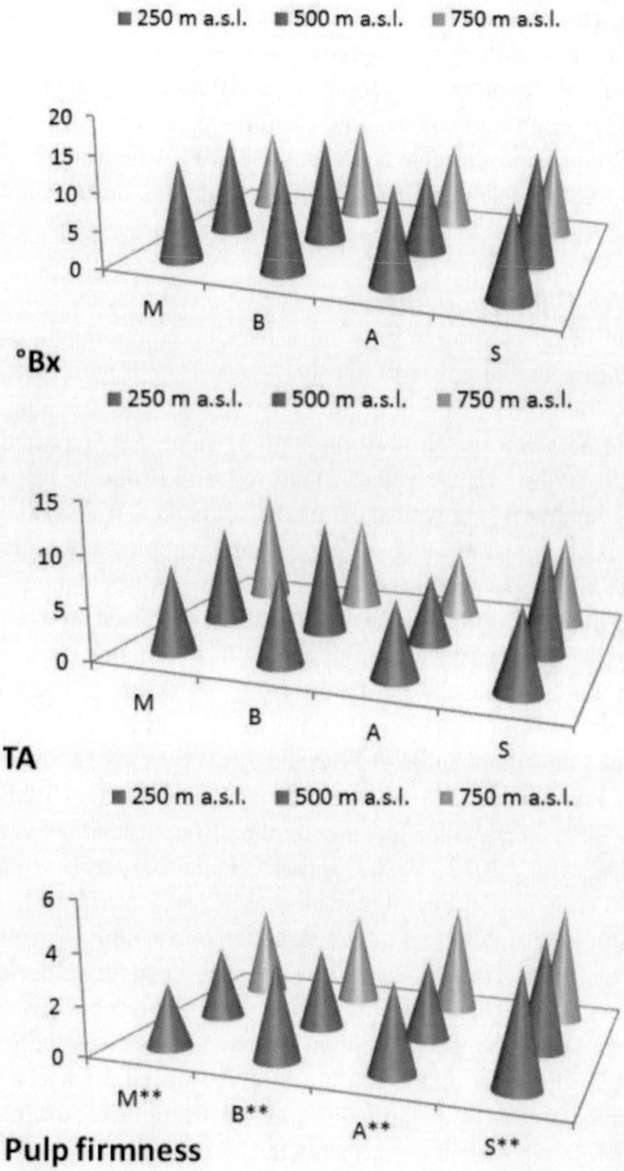

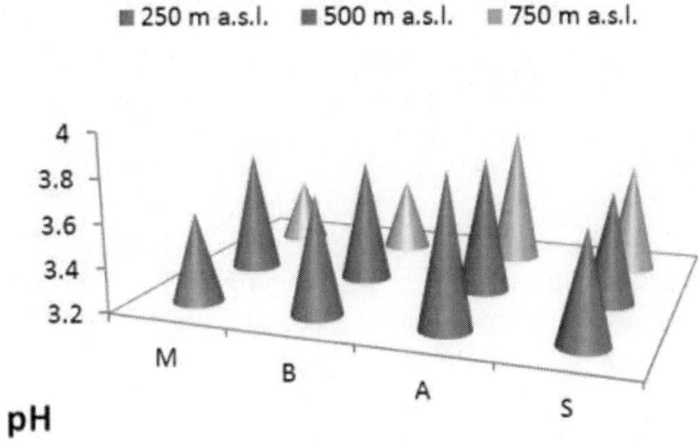

Figure 4. Physico-chemical parameters of the fruits of the four *Pescabivona* landraces collected at the three different altitudes. Values are expressed as the mean of three replicates. TA: titratable acidity (expressed as malic acid meq/100 g). Pulp firmness is expressed as kg/cm^2. M: *Murtiddara*; B: *Bianca*; A: *Agostina*; S: *Settembrina*. ANOVA: $^{**}p \leq 0.01$; $^{*}p \leq 0.05$ (adapted from Vasile Simone et al., 2014).

3.1.3. Organic Acids and Sugars Determination

Citric and malic acid were the most abundant organic acids (Figure 5), with a prevalence of the latter over the former. In particular, citric acid showed statistically significant differences among landraces, while malic acid among altitudes. Quinic acid and succinic acid did not show significant contents (Montevecchi et al., 2012; Vasile Simone et al., 2014).

The most abundant sugar was sucrose and the four landraces showed comparable levels of it (Figure 6). However, statistical analysis showed slight significant differences among the altitudes. In particular, the higher the altitudes the lower the accumulation of sucrose, probably because of the lower temperature that slows down the ripening process (Montevecchi et al., 2012; Vasile Simone et al., 2014). Very similar considerations can be made also for fructose and glucose, which were one order of magnitude less concentrated than the previous one (Figure 6).

3.1.4. Lactones Determination

The analysis of aromatic compounds was focused on four lactones: γ-decalattone, δ-decalactone, γ-dodecalactone, δ-dodecalactone, which represent the main volatile compounds of peach smell (Horvat et al., 1990). In particular, γ-decalattone and δ-decalactone are considered compounds of 'character impact' (Engel et al., 1988; Wang et al., 2009). γ-Lactones showed higher concentrations than the corresponding δ-lactones (Figure 7). To determine the contributions of individual lactones to peach aroma, odour activity value (OAV) was calculated as the ratio between the concentration of the lactones in the sample and their sensory threshold (Keith and Powers, 1968; Engel et al., 1988). γ-Lactones had highest concentrations and lowest thresholds of perception. γ-Dodecalactone showed statistically higher values among the landraces, while the relative variability did not allow discrimination among the altitudes. δ-Decalactone was of an order of magnitude lower than its γ-isomer, while δ-dodecalactone showed values below the sensory threshold or slightly above (Montevecchi et al., 2012; Vasile Simone et al., 2014).

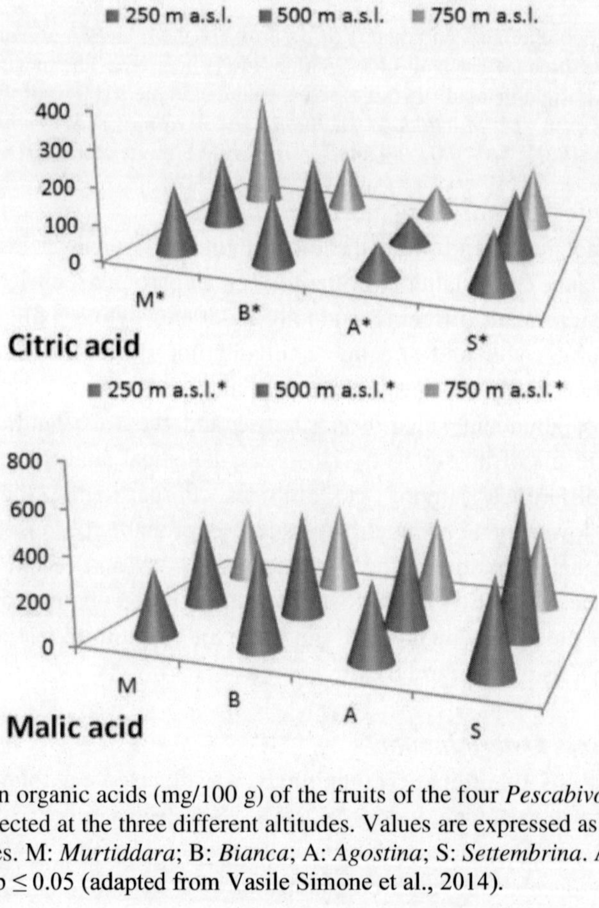

Figure 5. Main organic acids (mg/100 g) of the fruits of the four *Pescabivona* landraces collected at the three different altitudes. Values are expressed as the mean of three replicates. M: *Murtiddara*; B: *Bianca*; A: *Agostina*; S: *Settembrina*. ANOVA: $^{**}p \leq 0.01$; $^{*}p \leq 0.05$ (adapted from Vasile Simone et al., 2014).

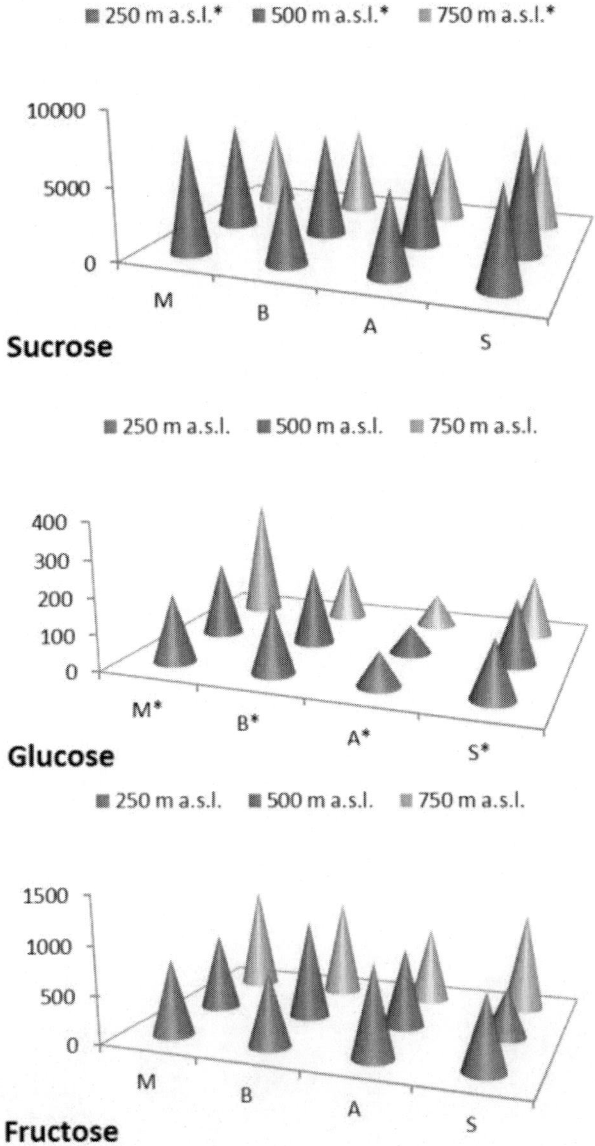

Figure 6. Main sugars (mg/100 g) of the fruits of the four *Pescabivona* landraces collected at the three different altitudes. Values are expressed as the mean of three replicates. M: *Murtiddara*; B: *Bianca*; A: *Agostina*; S: *Settembrina*.
ANOVA: **$p \leq 0.01$; *$p \leq 0.05$ (adapted from Vasile Simone et al., 2014).

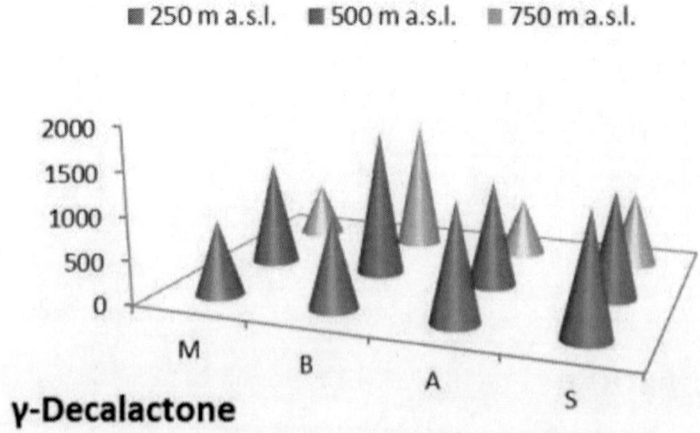
250 m a.s.l.
500 m a.s.l.
750 m a.s.l.
2000
1500
1000
500
0
M
B
A
S
γ-Decalactone

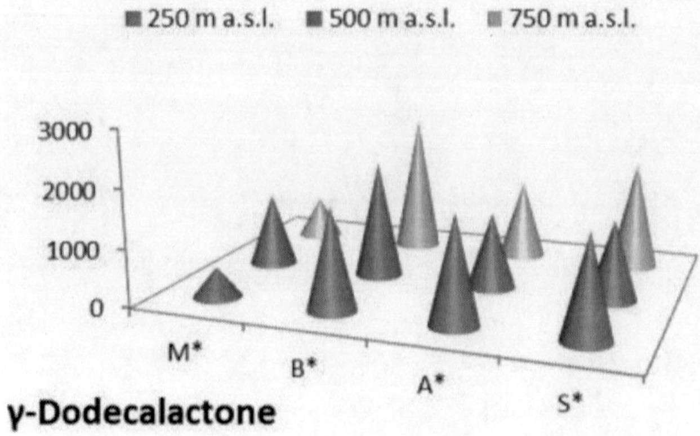
250 m a.s.l.
500 m a.s.l.
750 m a.s.l.
3000
2000
1000
0
M*
B*
A*
S*
γ-Dodecalactone

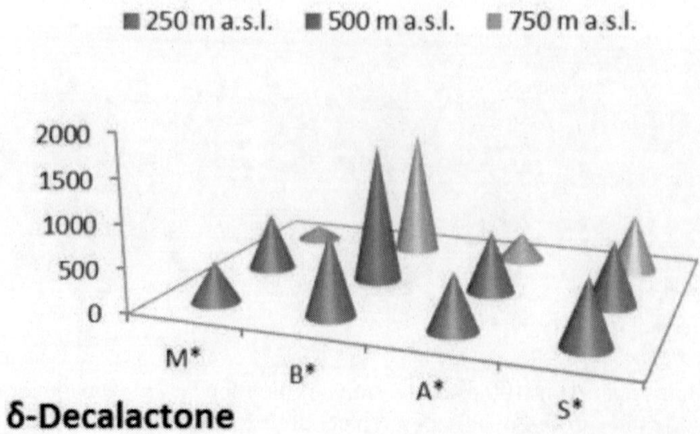
250 m a.s.l.
500 m a.s.l.
750 m a.s.l.
2000
1500
1000
500
0
M*
B*
A*
S*
δ-Decalactone

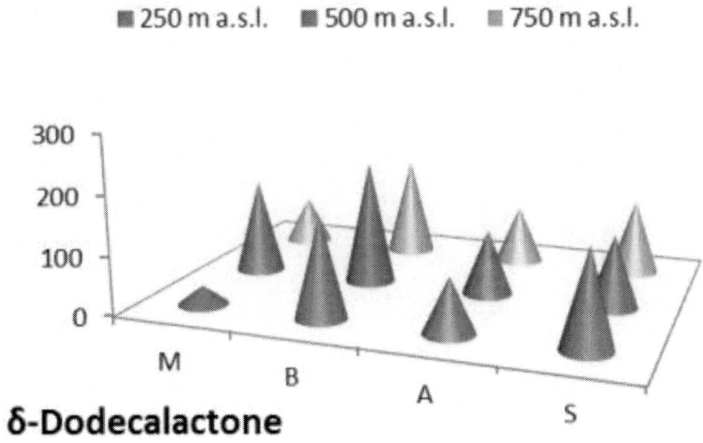

Figure 7. Lactones (μg/kg) of the fruits of the four *Pescabivona* landraces collected at the three different altitudes. Values are expressed as the mean of three replicates. M: *Murtiddara*; B: *Bianca*; A: *Agostina*; S: *Settembrina*. ANOVA: **$p \leq 0.01$; *$p \leq 0.05$ (adapted from Vasile Simone et al., 2014).

3.1.5. Phenolic and Antioxidant Capacity Measurement

For peaches, the antioxidant capacity is considered an important factor for quality assessment and for nutritional and nutraceutical properties (Infante et al., 2008). Phenolic compounds, in fact, are the main substances with reducing power that can counteract the free radicals (Dalla Valle et al., 2007). Flavan-3-ols and hydroxycinnamic acids (Figure 8) were determined. *Bianca*, followed by *Settembrina*, showed the highest content of pulp flavan-3-ols, mainly at the intermediate altitude (500 m a.s.l.). *Bianca* was the landraecs with the highest hydroxycinnamic acids content, as well (Figure 8).

Similar considerations can be done also for peel phenolic content (Figure 8). Although the phenolic determination was semi-quantitative, it was remarkable that *Bianca* contained, on average, a statistically higher amount of these substances (Montevecchi et al., 2012; Vasile Simone et al., 2014).

The data showed statistically significant differences among landraces for the antioxidant capacity. *Bianca* was confirmed as the cv. with highest antioxidant capacity for both peel and pulp (Figure 9), while the lowest values were observed for *Agostina* (Montevecchi et al., 2012; Vasile Simone et al., 2014).

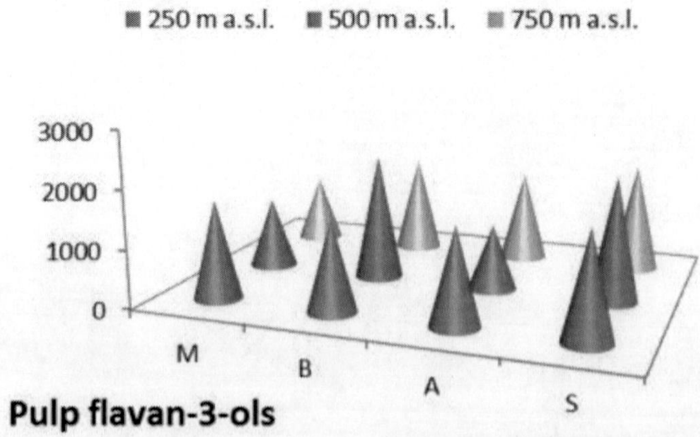
250 m a.s.l.
500 m a.s.l.
750 m a.s.l.
3000
2000
1000
0
M
B
A
S
Pulp flavan-3-ols

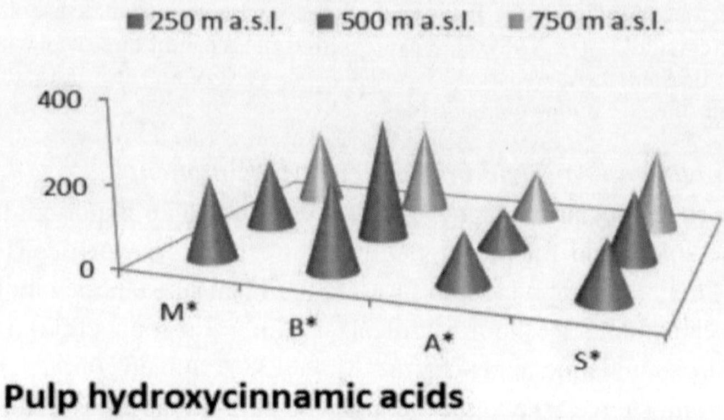
250 m a.s.l.
500 m a.s.l.
750 m a.s.l.
400
200
0
M*
B*
A*
S*
Pulp hydroxycinnamic acids

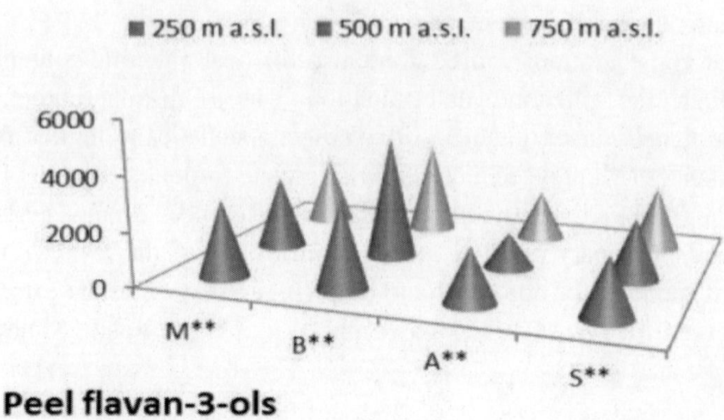
250 m a.s.l.
500 m a.s.l.
750 m a.s.l.
6000
4000
2000
0
M**
B**
A**
S**
Peel flavan-3-ols

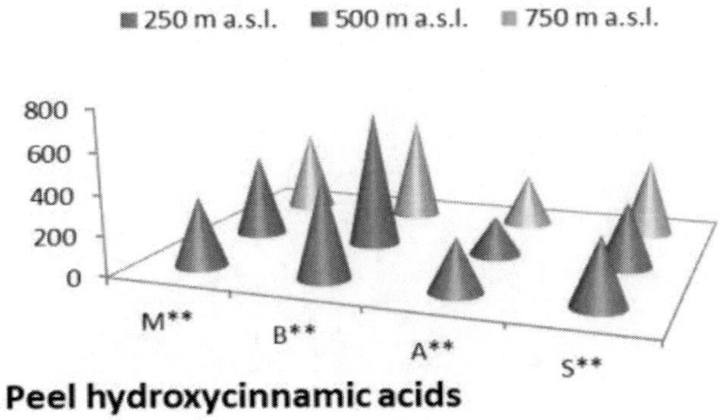

Figure 8. Flavan-3-ols (expressed as mg catechin equivalent/kg) and hydroxycinnamic acids (expressed as mg chlorogenic acid equivalent/kg) of pulp and peel of the fruits of the four *Pescabivona* landraces collected at the three different altitudes. Values are expressed as the mean of three replicates. M: *Murtiddara*; B: *Bianca*; A: *Agostina*; S: *Settembrina*. ANOVA: $^{**}p \leq 0.01$; $^{*}p \leq 0.05$ (adapted from Vasile Simone et al., 2014).

3.2. Sensory Analysis

The sliced fruits were all described by the panel as very fragrant and statistically significant differences (Figure 10) were not found for the intensity of smell (Montevecchi et al., 2013; Vasile Simone et al., 2014).

All the samples showed red veins near the stone, with the exception of *Murtiddara* whose fruits had a higher variability for this attribute. Among the descriptors of the structure, only the hardness did not allow to differentiate the samples. Juiciness was perceived high in *Murtiddara*, at intermediate level for *Bianca* and *Agostina*, while *Settembrina* was judged as the least juicy. Fibrousness got the highest scores for *Agostina* and intermediate scores for *Bianca* and *Settembrina*, whereas *Murtiddara* showed the lowest values (Montevecchi et al., 2013; Vasile Simone et al., 2014).

Settembrina peaches were assessed as the sweetest fruits, while the fruits of *Murtiddara*, despite having reached quite high scores, were judged as the least sweet. Sourness was perceived in all samples: *Murtiddara* peaches were the sourest fruits, Bianca and *Settembrina* were described with intermediate sourness values, while *Agostina* was the least sour. Bitterness was slightly perceived only for *Bianca*, showing statistically significant difference for this descriptor (Montevecchi et al., 2013; Vasile Simone et al., 2014).

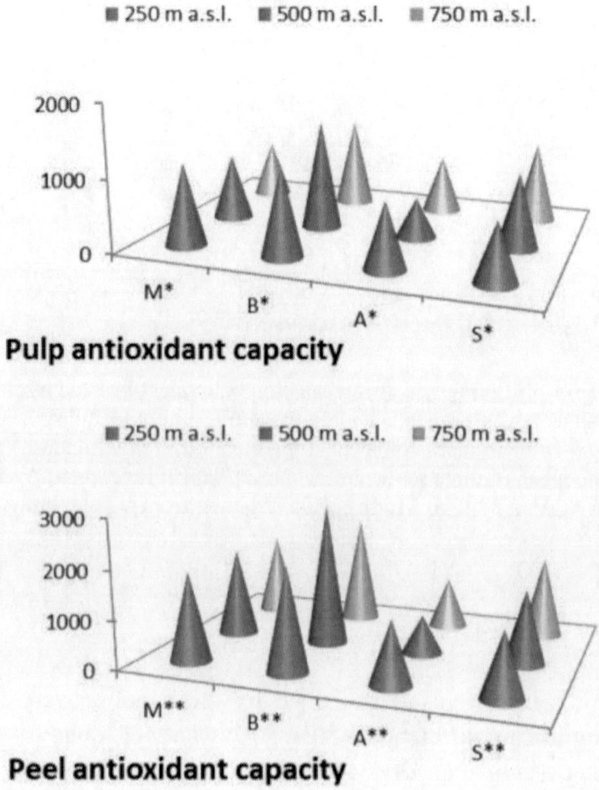

Figure 9. Antioxidant capacity (expressed as mg vitamin C equivalent/kg fresh peach) of pulp and peel of the fruits of the four *Pescabivona* landraces collected at the three different altitudes. Values are expressed as the mean of three replicates. M: *Murtiddara*; B: *Bianca*; A: *Agostina*; S: *Settembrina*. ANOVA: $^{**}p \leq 0.01$; $^{*}p \leq 0.05$ (adapted from Vasile Simone et al., 2014).

For *Settembrina*, peach aroma was perceived more intense than *Bianca*, and the other two landraces got intermediate evaluations.

The panel also provided a score related to the overall liking of the four landraces. *Settembrina* was the most appreciated, followed closely by *Agostina*, while *Murtiddara* and *Bianca* were the landraces less liked, albeit they obtained medium-high scores (Montevecchi et al., 2013; Vasile Simone et al., 2014).

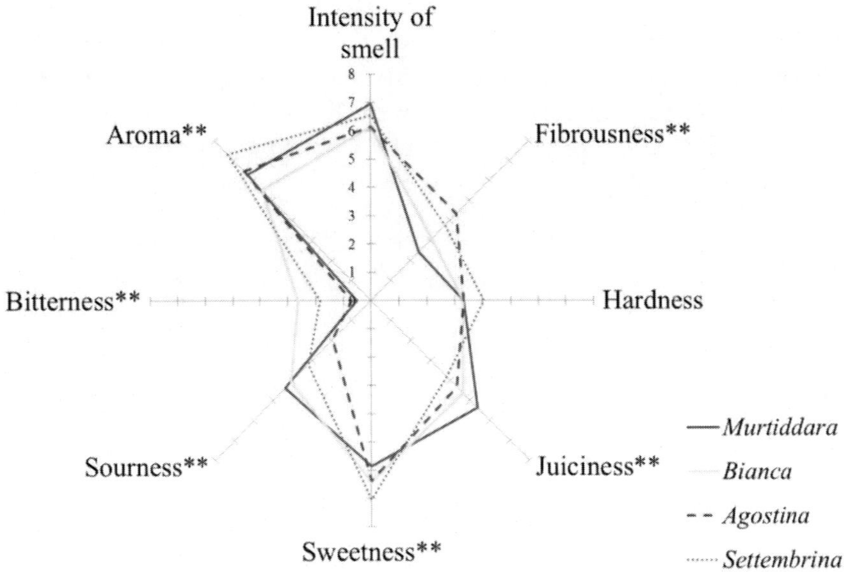

Figure 10. Comparison among sensory profiles of *Pescabivona* landraces ANOVA: $**p \leq 0.01$.

The evaluation of the whole fruit was carried out to provide a more complete description and to allow the judges the opportunity to deepen their knowledge on this kind of peach. The description of the whole fruit was performed at the end of each sensory session to reduce the possible influence of the whole fruit appearance on the sensory evaluation of the sliced fruits. The shape of the fruits was described as spheroidal, except *Bianca* that was indicated as oblate-spheroidal. The peel ground colour was described as white-green for *Agostina*, yellow-green for *Murtiddara* and *Bianca*, and white for *Settembrina*. The intensity of the smell was perceived high in *Murtiddara* and *Bianca*, whereas the other two landraces showed a more variable description. Anyhow, most of the judges indicated all the fruits as markedly fragrant (Montevecchi et al., 2013; Vasile Simone et al., 2014).

Recently, *Settembrina* was proved to be suitable for processing into fresh-cut products because it retains its physico-chemical (lowest degree of the browning index) and sensory (peach odor, visual appearance, crunchiness scores, and overall liking) characteristics better than the other landraces (Allegra et al., 2015).

Table 1. Comparison among the qualitative features of *Pescabivona* landraces (average values of the three altitudes) with the most common white flesh peach cvs. Data from the MiPAAF-Regioni project "Lists of variety orientation of fruit trees" (www.listevarietali.it) were used. SSC = soluble solid content; TA = titratable acidity (adapted from Vasile Simone et al., 2014)

Cultivar e maturazione	SSC (°Bx)	TA (meq/100 g)	SSC/TA	Percentage of red (%)	Pulp firmness*
Early ripening					
Alexandra	10.7	4.5	35.5	70	Medium
Crizia	12.1	9	20.1	65	High
Hermione	15.6	9.9	23.5	80	Low
Iris Rosso	11.2	9.5	17.6	85	Medium
Primerose	10.2	10.4	14.7	85	Medium
White Crest	9.0	9.7	13.8	70	Low
Pescabivona Murtiddara	13.0	9.9	19.6	43	Medium
Intermediate ripening					
Benedicte	12.1	16.6	10.9	55	Medium
Greta	12.9	11.8	16.3	80	Medium/high
Maria Rosa	11.9	9.6	18.6	70	Medium
Maria Bianca	14.0	11.3	18.6	55	Medium/high
Pescabivona Bianca	14.4	9.8	21.0	25	Medium/high
Late ripening					
Maria Delizia	12.8	10.0	19.2	50	Medium/high
Regina Bianca	13.0	8.5	22.8	60	Medium
Regina di Londa	13.5	9.4	21.4	25	Medium
Cultivar e maturazione	SSC (°Bx)	TA (meq/100 g)	SSC/TA	Percentage of red (%)	Pulp firmness*
Tendresse	14.0	14.1	14.8	80	Medium
Maria Angela	14.6	11.7	18.6	50	Medium
Douceur	15.5	5.0	46.2	40	Medium
Gladys	12.5	15.4	13.0	50	Medium/high
Pescabivona Agostina	12.3	6.9	26.3	33	Medium/high
Pescabivona Settembrina	13.3	9.4	20.8	30	High

The average values for pulp firmness were converted to a judgment according with what proposed by MiPAAF-Regioni "Lists of variety orientation of fruit trees" (www.listevarietali.it).

3.3. Comparison with Main cvs.

The data collected in the Italian MiPAAF-Regioni project (www.listevarietali.it) were used to compare *Pescabivona* landraces with the main white flesh peach cvs. that have similar fruit traits and ripening time.

All fruits of *Pescabivona* landraces showed medium-high values for SSC in comparison with the other cvs. On the contrary, TA presented data in line with the other cvs. or even lower (Table 1). These concomitant factors explain the high values of SSC/TA for *Pescabivona* and these data are correlated with the sensory analysis results (Vasile Simone et al., 2014).

The percentage of red over colour showed values, on average, lower than 50% for all *Pescabivona* landraces, unlike most of the cvs. reported in the cited list that exceeded 50% and in many cases even 70%.

For *Murtiddara* and *Bianca*, pulp firmness was consistent with that of the other cvs., while for *Agostina* and especially for *Settembrina*, the data showed a higher pulp firmness, on average. These data has a greater significance when related to the corresponding SSC to TA ratios. The fruits showed, in fact, SSC to TA ratios typical for 'ready-to-eat' fruits simultaneously with a pulp firmness typical of a commercial ripening (Vasile Simone et al., 2014).

Conclusion

The results of these studies showed the high quality of *Pescabivona* fruits, highlighting several proper features with respect to the most common white flesh peach cvs., together with some traits typical of the old varieties. In particular, the limited extension of red over colour recalls the old white peaches, but for this reason it should not diminish the appreciation by consumers.

Noteworthy is the high sugar content of the early variety, character that should be used by breeders to improve the standard of cvs. of the same ripening time, which generally lack for this aspect.

Certainly, the main peculiar feature of these Sicilian cvs. is the persistence of pulp firmness even at levels of consumption ripening, especially for late ripening landraces. In fact, in a period of the year in which peach quality generally lowers, the high pulp firmness reduces the risk of bruises and browning and becomes an uncommon chance to taste fruits at physiological maturity consistent with an appreciable sensory profile. In addition, these conditions provide the sensory quality that usually is found in fruits nearing the end of their shelf-life, as well as assure a good management of post-harvesting.

REFERENCES

Allegra, A., Barone, E., Inglese, P., Todaro, A., and Sortino, G. 2015. "Variability of sensory profile and quality characteristics for 'Pesca di Bivona'and 'Pesca di Leonforte'peach (*Prunus persica* Batsch) fresh-cut slices during storage." *Postharvest Biology and Technology* 110:61–69.

Bassi, D., and Piagnani, M.C. 2008. "Morfologia e fenologia" in *Il pesco*. Series "Coltura e Cultura." 1–17. Milan: Bayer Crop Science S.r.l.

Bassi, D., Liverani L., Giovannini D., Foschi S., and Lama M. 2010a. "Il miglioramento genetico del pesco, nuove tipologie ed extra-stagionalità di pesche e nettarine." *Italus Hortus* 17(5):23–28.

Bassi, D., Sansavini, S., Tartarini, S., Dondini, L., Foschi, S., Vecchietti, A., and Missere, D. 2010b. "Il progetto MAS.PES a co-finanziamento pubblico-privato per il miglioramento genetico di albicocco e pesco assistito da tecniche di biologia molecolare." *Italus Hortus* 17(5):29–30.

Bassi, D., and Foschi, S. 2013. "Trends in apricot and peach industries in Italy." Proceedings of the IV Conference "Innovation in fruit growing," Belgrade, Serbia, 49–73, February 11.

Billmeyer, F. W., and Saltzman, M. 1981. "Describing colour." In *Principles of colour technology* (2nd ed.) edited by F. W. Billmeyer, and M. Saltzman, 31–74. New York (USA): Wiley and Sons.

Cannella, C. 2008. "Aspetti nutrizionali" in *Il pesco*. Series "Coltura e Cultura." 76–81. Milan: Bayer Crop Science S.r.l.

Cantín, C. M., Gogorcena, Y., and Moreno, M. A. 2010. "Phenotypic diversity and relationships of fruit quality traits in peach and nectarine [*Prunus persica* (L.) Batsch] breeding progenies." *Euphytica* 171:211–226.

Caruso, T. 1982. "La pesca di Bivona." *L'Informatore Agrario* 38:21439–21440.

Caruso, T., Marchese, A., Monte, M., Sottile, F., Bottalico, G., Cartabellotta, D., Di Martino, V., and Marrone, G. 2005. "Il germoplasma autoctono del pesco [*P. persica* (L.) Batsch] in Sicilia: aspetti fenologici, morfologici e molecolari." Proceedings of the VII National Conference on Biodiversity "L'agrobiodiversità per la qualificazione delle filiere produttive," Catania, Italy, 43, March 30 – April 2.

Castellari, L. 2002. "I caratteri della qualità. Pianeta pesca. Qualità e sicurezza per il consumatore." *Il Divulgatore* 3–4.

Chinnici, F., Spinabelli, U., Riponi, C., and Amati, A. 2005. "Optimization of the determination of organic acids and sugars in fruit juices by ion-exclusion liquid chromatography." *Journal of Food Composition and Analysis* 18:121–130.

Cusumano, G. 2009. "La pesca di Bivona verso l'IGP." *Rivista di Frutticoltura e di Ortofloricoltura* 71(4):82–83.

Dalla Valle, A. Z., Mignani, I., Spinardi, A., Galvano, F., and Ciappellano, S. 2007. "The antioxidant profile of three different peaches cultivars (*Prunus persica*) and their short-term effect on antioxidant status in human." *European Food Research and Technology* 225:167–172.

Dirlewanger, E., Moing, A., Rothan, C., Svanella, L., Pronier, V., Guye, A., Plomion, C., and Monet, R. 1999. "Mapping QTLs controlling fruit quality in peach (*Prunus persica* (L.) Batsch)." *TAG Theoretical and Applied Genetics* 98:18–31.

Engel, K. H., Flath, R. A., Buttery, R. G., Mon, T. R., Ramming, D. W., and Teranishi, R. 1988. "Investigation of volatile constituents in nectarines. 1. Analytical and sensory characterization of aroma components in some nectarine cultivars." *Journal of Agricultural and Food Chemistry* 36:549–553.

Esti, M., Messia, M. C., Sinesio, F., Nicotra, A., Conte, L., La Notte, E., and Palleschi, G. 1997. "Quality evaluation of peaches and nectarines by electrochemical and multivariate analyses: relationships between analytical measurements and sensory attributes." *Food Chemistry* 60(4):659–666.

Fideghelli, C. 2008. "Allevamento e potatura" in *Il pesco*. Series "Coltura e Cultura." Milan: Bayer Crop Science S.r.l.

Fideghelli, C. 2012. "La situazione italiana nel contesto internazionale." *Rivista di Frutticoltura e di Ortofloricoltura* 7-8:20–26.

Génard, M., and Bruchou, C. 1992. "Multivariate analysis of within-tree factors accounting for the variation of peach fruit quality." *Scientia Horticulturae* 52:37–51.

G.U.R.I. 2013. Gazzetta Ufficiale della Repubblica Italiana n. 125 of 05/30/2013. http://www.gazzettaufficiale.it/atto/vediMenuHTML?atto.dataPubblicazioneGazzetta=2013-05-30&atto.codiceRedazionale=13A04570&tipoSerie=serie_generale&tipoVigenza=originario.

O.J.E.U. 2014. Official Journal of the European Union C 103/13 of 08/04/2014. http://eur-lex.europa.eu/legal-content/EN/TXT/HTML/?uri=CELEX:52014XC0408%2801%29&from=ET.

Giovannini, D., and Liverani A., 2014. "Il breeding del pesco, un percorso secolare ricco di nuove tipologie di frutti." *Rivista di Frutticoltura* 7-8:8–14.

Horvat, R. J., Chapman, G. W., Jr., Robertson, J. A., Meredith, F. I., Scorza, R., Callahan, A. M., and Morgens, P. 1990. "Comparison of the volatile compounds from several commercial peach cultivars." *Journal of Agricultural and Food Chemistry* 38:234–237.

Iglesias, I. 2013. "Peach production in Spain: Current situation and trends, from production to consumption." Proceedings of the IV Conference "Innovation in fruit growing," Belgrade, Serbia, 75–98, February 11.

Infante, R., Martínez-Gómez, P., and Predieri, S. 2008. "Quality oriented fruit breeding: Peach [*Prunus persica* (L.) Batsch]." *Journal of Food, Agriculture and Environment* 6:342–356.

Keith, E. S., and Powers, J. J. 1968. "Determination of flavor threshold levels and subthreshold, additive, and concentration effects." *Journal of Food Science*, 33:213–218.

Layne, D. R., and Bassi, D. 2008. The peach: botany, production and uses. Wallingford, UK: CABI.

Liverani, A. 2008. "Miglioramento genetico" in *Il pesco*. Series "Coltura e Cultura." 306–339. Milan: Bayer Crop Science S.r.l.

Liverani, A., Giovannini, D., Brandi, F., Merli, M., Pellegrino, S., and Berra, L. 2006. "Nuove pesche a polpa bianca dalla ricerca genetica pubblica." *Frutticoltura* 9:60–63.

Liverani, A., Predieri, S., Gatti, E., and Versari, N. 2008. "Cosa vogliono i consumatori? Test sensoriali sulle nuove tipologie di prodotto." *Rivista di Frutticoltura e di Ortofloricoltura* 7-8:20–25.

Marchese, A., Tobutt, K., Campisi, G., Cartabellotta, D., Di Martino, V., Marrone, G., and Caruso, T. 2006. "Il germoplasma autoctono del pesco [*Prunus persica* (L.) Batsch]. Sicilia: aspetti fenologici, morfologici e molecolari." *Italus Hortus* 13:118–122.

Montevecchi G., Vasile Simone G., Masino F., Bignami C., and Antonelli A. 2012. "Physical and chemical characterization of Pescabivona, a Sicilian white flesh peach cultivar [*Prunus persica* (L.) Batsch]." *Food Research International* 45(1):123–131.

Montevecchi, G., Vasile Simone, G., Mellano, M. G., Masino, F., and Antonelli, A. 2013. "Sensory characterization of the four Pescabivona landraces, white flesh peaches [*Prunus persica* (L.) Batsch] and correlation with physical and chemical parameters." *Fruits* 68(3):195–207.

Pedrieri, S., and Rapparini, F. 2008. "Aromi e sapori" in *Il pesco*. Series "Coltura e Cultura." 306–339. Milan: Bayer Crop Science S.r.l.

Pérez, A. G., Olías, R., Espada, J., Olías, J. M., and Sanz, C. 1997. "Rapid determination of sugars, non volatile acids, and ascorbic acid in strawberry and other fruits." *Journal of Agricultural and Food Chemistry* 45:3545–3549.

Re, R., Pellegrini, N., Proteggente, A., Pannala, A., Yang, M., and Rice-Evans, C. A. 1999. "Antioxidant activity applying an improved ABTS radical cation decolorization assay." *Free Radical Biology and Medicine* 26:1231–1237.

Tavarini, S., Degl'Innocenti, E., Remorini, D., Massai, R., and Guidi L. 2008. "Preliminary characterisation of peach cultivars for their antioxidant capacity." *International Journal of Food Science and Technology* 43:810–815.

Vasile Simone, G., Montevecchi, G., Masino, F., Mellano, M. G., Bignami, C., and Antonelli, A. 2014. "Pescabivona: caratterizzazione e specificità dei frutti nell'ambito del regime di qualità IGP." *Industrie Alimentari* 53(550):15–24.

Wang, Y., Yang, C., Li, S., Yang, L., Wang, Y., Zhao, J., and Jiang, Q. 2009. "Volatile characteristics of 50 peaches and nectarines evaluated by HP-SPME with GC-MS." *Food Chemistry* 116:356–364.

www.listevarietali.it Liste varietali di Pesco a polpa bianca.

INDEX

D

G

H

I

N

O

P

Q

R

S

T

U

V

W

X

Y

Z